Disasters, Public Health Emergencies, and Crisis Response

Cognella Series on
Public and Community Health Nursing

Disasters, Public Health Emergencies, and Crisis Response

Anita Finkelman, MSN, RN

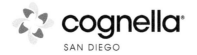

cognella
SAN DIEGO

Bassim Hamadeh, CEO and Publisher
Amanda Martin, Publisher
Amy Smith, Senior Project Editor
Rachel Kahn, Production Editor
Jess Estrella, Senior Graphic Designer
Kylie Bartolome, Licensing Coordinator
Natalie Piccotti, Director of Marketing
Kassie Graves, Vice President of Editorial
Jamie Giganti, Director of Academic Publishing

This book is designed to provide educational information and motivation to our readers. It is sold with the understanding that the publisher is not engaged to render any type of psychological, legal, diet, health, exercise or any other kind of professional advice. The content of each chapter or reading is the sole expression and opinion of its author, and not necessarily that of the publisher. No warranties or guarantees are expressed or implied by the publisher's choice to include any of the content in this volume. Neither the publisher nor the individual author(s) shall be liable for any physical, psychological, emotional, financial, or commercial damages, including, but not limited to, special, incidental, consequential or other damages. Our views and rights are the same: You are responsible for your own choices, actions, and results and for seeking relevant topical advice from trained professionals.

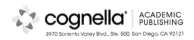

cognella® | ACADEMIC PUBLISHING
3970 Sorrento Valley Blvd., Ste. 500, San Diego, CA 92121

This project is dedicated to all the students who have taught me during my years of professional practice in clinical and academic settings. I also recognize the nurses who have provided care daily during a difficult time of a pandemic, treating all equally in all settings and communities, and with special thoughts for those nurses who experienced illness and lost their lives as they worked to improve the health of their communities.

Contents

ACTIVE LEARNING

This book has interactive activities available to complement your reading.

Your instructor may have customized the selection of activities available for your unique course. Please check with your professor to verify whether your class will access this content through the Cognella Active Learning portal (http://active.cognella.com) or through your home learning management system.

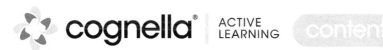 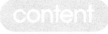

Preface

D ue to our experience with the COVID-19 pandemic, nurses have confronted many new issues as well as questioned the quality of past health care delivery and education. This has impacted and will continue to impact all aspects of health care delivery globally, and this includes nursing. This content focuses on improving public and community health and emphasizes the need for the nursing profession and health care delivery to recognize that we must do more to make this area of health care as integral to health care delivery as is acute care. Nursing students are eager to "get into *real nursing*" in the hospital; however, with our experiences with COVID-19, we now should be more aware that public and community health is critical for the health of individuals, families, populations, communities, individual countries, and the global population and impacts all aspects of life. We also recognize more that this is not a simple area of health care, which has long been a common view. Public and community health is influenced by equity and justice, culture policies, governments, laws, ethics, economics, and much more. In addition, this information changes quickly, requiring nurses to be aware of changes and new information and then integrate this information into public and community health practice. This is not easy to accomplish, and it is complex due to the need to consider a broad variety of factors, social determinants of health. Population health and vulnerable populations have an impact on the overall health status of communities and countries. This requires attention to health equity and recognition that we have serious disparities in health delivery and outcomes that must be addressed in all health care settings. The nursing profession has acknowledged this through its recent standards and ethics; statements about racism, discrimination, health equity, and disparities; and strategies to improve population health. There is now recognition that we need more student experiences in a variety of health care settings in addition to acute care to prepare a nursing workforce that can also practice effectively in public and community health. Major reports from experts recognize the need for change must be addressed: *The Future of Nursing 2020–2030: Charting a Path to Achieving Health Equity* (National Academy of Medicine, 2021), the third report in a series on the future of nursing, indicates that nursing education must consider and integrate content and clinical experiences that address social determinants of health (SDOH), health equity, and population health, which are not currently integrated in curricula. Students need clinical experiences with different people, varied life experiences, and cultural values. This all requires greater nursing leadership and engagement in continuous quality improvement in public and community health.

This guide addresses some of these issues by focusing on disaster and public health emergencies. Nurses are active in these situations and during all phases of activity. Emergency management needs to consider diversity and equity to ensure that all who need help receive help during disasters and public health emergencies. This content discusses some of these factors and their implications for preparedness, response, and recovery. Vulnerable populations are discussed as well as their special needs during these times. There are multiple stakeholders that are involved during disasters and public health emergencies including government, nongovernmental agencies or organizations, humanitarian organizations, and businesses. These stakeholders are described in this content. The nursing profession is very involved in engaging in this topic to ensure that communities receive the care they need during these critical times.

Acknowledgments

I thank my family for their support of my writing and professional endeavors over many years: Fred, Shoshannah, and Deborah—and especially my grandson, Matanel Yizhar, who teaches me daily that learning is constant as well as caring. Thank you to Amanda Martin, a long-time publishing colleague who reached out to me to connect again to develop this project. The Cognella team cannot be praised enough for their professionalism and creativity: Amy Smith for directing editing guidance and keeping me on track; Dani Grandsher, Haley Brown, and all the others who helped with the development of methods supporting creative student engagement in learning and effective faculty resources; Jeannine Rees for guiding production; Natalie Piccotti, who leads the marketing initiative; and so many others who have helped on this project behind the scenes.

Disasters, Public Health Emergencies, and Crisis Response

Learning Outcomes

1. Formulate a description of disasters and public health emergencies, crisis response, and the importance of equity, disparities, and social determinants of health.

2. Compare and contrast disasters and public health emergencies.

3. Compare and contrast the roles of the government, non-profit and humanitarian organizations, and the private sector during times of disasters and public health emergencies.

4. Critique the use of emergency management during disasters and public health emergencies.

5. Summarize how disaster preparedness should be applied, including process and structure, the three C's, funding, and resources.

6. Differentiate how communities and vulnerable populations experience disasters and public health emergencies.

7. Critique some of the common responses to disasters and public health emergencies and how these responses impact outcomes for individuals, families, populations, and communities.

8. Apply nursing roles and interventions to disasters, public health emergencies, and crisis response.

9. Formulate a summary statement highlighting key points about disasters, public health emergencies, and crisis response.

Key Terms

Community emergency response team	First responder	Protection
Disaster	Frequency	Quarantine
Displaced person	Incident action plan	Recovery
Emergency management	Isolation	Refugee
Emergency medical services	Mitigation	Relief
Emergency operations center	Posttraumatic stress disorder (PTSD)	Resilience
	Preparedness	Response
	Prevention	Triage

Introduction

This guide focuses on disasters, public health emergencies, and crisis response; all impact public and community health. Disasters and public health emergencies can affect any area or the country without regard to political, governmental jurisdictions, levels of government, religion, age of population, or geographical boundaries. A disaster or public health emergency is a critical time for collaboration and coordination across boundaries and with different organizations, public and private. The key goal is the health, safety, and welfare of the community and its populations. This guide's content provides an overview of the topic and examines approaches taken to prepare and respond and the roles and responsibilities of nurses during disasters and public health emergencies.

Overview: Disasters, Public Health Emergencies, and Crisis Response

Disasters and public health emergencies are not new. They have impacted individual states, countries, and the world. The COVID-19 pandemic represents a global public health emergency, though in this guide the content focuses on the United States and its experiences with disasters and public health emergencies, including the most current one, COVID-19.

> In the last decade, 2.6 billion people globally have been upended by earthquakes, floods, wildfires and other natural disasters. And now, the global coronavirus pandemic has killed more than 3 million people worldwide. All these crises disproportionately affect people of color, those with low incomes, those experiencing housing insecurity, and those with limited access to health care and transportation, ultimately exacerbating health disparities. (National Academy of Medicine [NAM], 2021a)

How did the United States recognize the need for an organized approach to public health emergency? NAM recognized the importance of public health preparedness and response and developed a report on this topic in 2020. The federal government identified public health and preparedness as a concern in 1946. World War II was concluding, and the United States was experiencing many cases of malaria. The Public Health Service (PHS) was created to assist during infectious disease outbreaks, particularly annual influenza outbreaks and then other infectious diseases. This led to the establishment of the Communicable Disease Center (CDC) as part of the U.S. Department of Health and Human Services (HHS). In 1992 the name was changed to the Centers for Disease Control and Prevention, though it is still referred to as the CDC. The CDC assisted several states through their state health departments in infectious disease control, and in the 1990s new risks arose, such as bioterrorism, which required public heath preparedness. Today, these risks increase with incidents that have required emergency management such as the Boston Marathon bombing and other incidents. The NAM report noted that over the years funding for research expanded in this area, but problems with effective preparedness and response continue. Evidence-based practice (EBP) is now a critical element in health care; however, more is needed in public health—evidence to support interventions and other needs during public health emergencies. This report focuses on four of the CDC's 15 preparedness and response capabilities: (a) community preparedness activating a public health emergency operations center; (b) emergency operations coordination, communicating public health alerts and guidance; (c) information sharing, implementing quarantine when needed; and (d) nonpharmaceutical interventions. Nursing should be involved in developing research to address these issues.

Critical Factors Impacting Disasters, Public Health, Emergencies, and Crisis Response

There are many important factors of society that impact disasters and public health emergencies. Addressing these issues first will help to better understand these experiences and lead to more effective preparedness and responses. Public and community health are critical aspects of a community's health care system. Public health functions and services are described in **Appendix A**. What do we need to consider about the community to better prepare and respond to these experiences that cause stress and loss to individuals, families, populations, and communities?

Social determinants of health (SDOH) must be considered when disasters and public health emergencies are assessed, and plans made to prevent or respond to them. Understanding the present condition of the community and populations helps to understand needs and response. SDOH are "the conditions in the environments where people are born, live, learn, work, play, worship, and age that affect a wide range of health, functioning, and quality-of-life outcomes and risks" (HHS, Office of Disease Prevention and Health Promotion [ODPHP], 2022a). The five SDOH domains or categories are as follows:

- Economic stability
- Education access and quality
- Health care access and quality
- Neighborhood and built environment
- Social and community context

How do the SDOH impact a community? They are associated with health, safe housing, transportation, racism and discrimination, job opportunities, income, access to nutritious food, physical activities, air and water quality, education, language and literacy, and individual and community safety. How does this connect to disasters and public emergencies? If a community or a specific population is struggling with SDOH before a disaster then they enter the experience with less strength, and this could result in more complex outcomes for individuals, families, populations, and communities. For example, prior to the COVID-19 pandemic, which is a public health emergency, there were communities struggling with unemployment, civil unrest and criminal violence, poor health status, and inadequate access to health services, disparities, and other problems leading to a disproportionate impact on some vulnerable populations. This experience has put more attention on SDOH and on health equity (Robichaux & Sauerland, 2021).

Health equity has become a critical concern within the HHS, its agencies, and functions. "Healthcare inequity has always been a challenge across the U.S. The rate of disasters has increased over the years and the COVID-19 pandemic has ravaged the country, striking communities of color and other underserved populations especially hard. Healthcare professionals and emergency managers may benefit from a better understanding of the complex relationships that affect fair access to healthcare" and some of the definitions used by HHS agencies are (HHS, 2022a):

- The Health Resources and Services Administration (HRSA) defines health equity as "the absence of disparities or avoidable differences among socioeconomic and demographic groups or geographical areas in health status and health outcomes such as disease, disability, or mortality."
- The Office of Minority Health defines health equity as "the attainment of the highest level of health for all people. Achieving health equity requires valuing everyone equally with focused and ongoing societal

efforts to address avoidable inequalities, historical and contemporary injustices, and the elimination of health and healthcare disparities."

Equity is a part of all aspects of health care and must also be considered in all actions taken during a disaster or public health emergency and post-incident responses. To recognize this importance even the Federal Emergency Management Agency (FEMA) has an office of equal rights (DHS, FEMA, 2022a).

A current major goal in health care services is to reduce health disparities or differences in health outcomes among different populations, also a concern during disasters and public health emergencies. We want to ensure that all have equal opportunity for health and safety even during times of crisis. We know that urbanization and population growth in some areas increase risks, for example a major storm will then impact more people in these areas and may make it more difficult to reach all who need help in a timely manner.

> Yet widening social inequalities have left vulnerable/marginalized groups particularly susceptible to these extreme events. Structural racism, which manifests in both inequitable locational proximity to hazards and stark disparities in the resources people can use to respond to disaster, among other vulnerabilities, is at the root of racialized disaster impacts and must be dismantled through a broad range of antiracist social and economic policies. (Raker et al., 2020)

Health equity is a necessary element for effective preparedness (Nelson, 2021). COVID-19 as a national (and global) public health emergency makes it clear that some populations experience disparities, many prior to the pandemic, but also during the pandemic. SDOH, race, and ethnicity were not sufficiently considered in efforts to mitigate and respond to the pandemic. This has happened in other disasters, for example, during times of extreme weather such as a hurricane when people with limited funds could not buy supplies needed to protect their homes and businesses and did not have insurance to cover damage, lacked transportation to leave an unsafe area quickly, or had limited funds to buy extra food supplies, rent hotel or other temporary housing, and so on (Nelson, 2021).

An example of a weather-related disaster with disparities implications that was localized in that it only directly impacted several states and one city and state more was Hurricane Katrina, which in 2005 made a major hit on New Orleans and Louisiana. This disaster emphasized that populations that experience disparities prior to a hurricane—economic, housing, health services—are even more vulnerable when they experience major disruptions and loss during a disaster (Quinn, 2006). This disaster revealed a major social problem in this community that had long-term consequences. Many people could not evacuate, putting them at high risk during the storm. The poverty level was high in the community, and the non-White population felt that prior to the hurricane they had been treated differently from the White population, and this was exacerbated during the storm and recovery. Racial and minority groups felt that their government on all levels did not provide effective assistance during all the phases of the disaster. Many residents had to leave the location temporarily, and some never returned. This was a burden to other states who needed to provide services to these displaced persons. This type of experience has not just been experienced by the people of New Orleans during a disaster, as the experience shook the United States when media coverage illustrated the major disparities and loss. News coverage was high and with access to the internet and social media, information can be shared quickly, and in this case, there were many examples of problems and lack of effective responses.

Another example of a public health emergency that was directly impacted by inequities was the Flint, Michigan, water crisis, where the community experienced years of exposure to lead in their drinking water beginning in 2014. When changes were made in the water system the local government did not take the steps necessary to ensure safe water for all. This resulted in problems such as high lead levels, which was dangerous for all but particularly for children. This led to problems for children such as hyperactivity, slowed growth, lower IQ, anemia, and cardiovascular problems, and in adults reproductive problems (Environmental Protection Agency [EPA], 2022). There were 12 known deaths associated with the environmental problem. During a critical point water had to be brought in for the community, requiring large supplies of water and distribution methods so that homes, businesses, and schools had safe water for drinking, cooking, cleaning, and personal hygiene. Many in the city experienced greater socioeconomic problems than prior to this water crisis. These problems are difficult to resolve and take time.

Disasters and Public Health Emergencies

Disasters and public health emergencies have different causes but both are difficult to reliably predict. Both require similar response structure and process and use of emergency management, which is discussed later in this content.

Disasters

Disasters are "serious disruptions to the functioning of a community that exceed its capacity to cope using its own resources. Disasters can be caused by natural, man-made and technological hazards, as well as various factors that influence the exposure and vulnerability of a community" (International Federation of Red Cross and Red Crescent Societies [IFRC], 2022a). Some examples of man-made disasters are wars, which lead to destruction of communities and infrastructure and put people at physical and psychological risk. There are also actions taken by people that may lead to disasters, such as deforestation, overgrazing of livestock, and other actions that negatively impact the land and then the ability to farm, or impact the air and water quality, and so on.

> Natural disasters include all types of severe weather, which have the potential to pose a significant threat to human health and safety, property, critical infrastructure, and homeland security. Natural disasters occur both seasonally and without warning, subjecting the nation to frequent periods of insecurity, disruption, and economic loss. (HHS, DHS, 2021a)

Examples are floods, winter storms, tornados, hurricanes, earthquakes, and wildfires. The IFRC (2022b) identifies several key natural hazards that can lead to disasters and public health emergencies:

- **Geophysical:** A hazard originating from solid earth (e.g., earthquakes, landslides and volcanic activity)
- **Hydrological:** Caused by the occurrence, movement, and distribution of water on earth (e.g., floods and avalanches)
- **Climatological:** Relating to the climate (e.g., droughts and wildfires)
- **Meteorological:** Relating to weather conditions (e.g., cyclones and storms)
- **Biological:** Caused by exposure to living organisms and their toxic substances or diseases they may carry (e.g., disease epidemics and insect/animal plagues)

Climate change is an important topic today that has social, health, economic, and political implications. Making changes requires governmental and business collaboration, and it is a global issue, as real improvement requires action from multiple countries. It impacts many people who struggle economically and may live in unhealthy environments. Climate change has resulted in major weather problems that lead to disasters such as floods, fires, extreme temperatures, and so on. Air and water quality lead to health problems or make health problems worse such as cardiac and respiratory conditions. Air pollution has no boundaries, but populations that already struggle with inequities may suffer more. These communities may have less resources and leadership to address the problems, making health inequities rooted in structural racism worse (Robert Wood Johnson Foundation [RWJF], 2021). This is a major problem, and in 2021, 42 countries' health care organizations agreed to reduce their emissions of greenhouse gases (Choi-Schagrin, 2021). The agreement includes countries that are low, medium, and high income. Why are health care organizations included in this type of decision? Health care activities account for almost 5% of the carbon dioxide emissions. At the recent global climate summit in 2021, public health was more important than in the past, probably due to the influence of the COVID-19 pandemic and recognition of major health problems caused by climate change. The summer of 2022 demonstrating the critical nature of climate change and increased problems globally impacting health, economics, agriculture, and food and water supplies.

There is considerable evidence that the environment directly affects health status and impacts quality of life, years of healthy life lived, and health disparities. An example of an environmental factor is poor air quality, which is associated with premature death, cancer, and long-term damage to respiratory and cardiovascular systems. There is much said about the risks of smoking on individuals, but a related factor is the risk of secondhand smoke that impacts people around smokers and may result in heart disease and lung cancer in nonsmoking adults; smoking also may cause or exacerbate asthma in children. Globally, nearly 25% of all deaths and the total disease burden can be attributed to environmental factors and are particularly dangerous for people who already have chronic health problems. For example, nearly 1 in 10 children and 1 in 12 adults in the United States have asthma, which is caused, triggered, and exacerbated by environmental factors such as air pollution and secondhand smoke (HHS, ODPHP, 2022b). Globally, more than 12 million people die annually due to unhealthy environments. To decrease health problems environmental pollutants in air, water, soil, food, and materials in homes and workplaces need to be reduced. Healthy People 2030 includes environmental health objectives, as did Healthy People 2020. The current Healthy People goal is to promote healthier environments to improve health (HHS, ODPHP, 2022c).

In January 2021, President Biden issued an executive order recognizing climate change as a climate crisis that threatens people and communities, public health, and the economy (The White House, 2021a). President Biden established a National Climate Task Force, noting that a clean energy approach is positive for all. The task force supports multiple approaches to deal with a variety of climate-related problems, for example, four in ten Americans live in a county that was impacted by a climate disaster last year. As climate-related extreme weather events increase in frequency and ferocity, the U.S. is taking bold steps to strengthen the nation's resilience to severe impacts climate change has on our communities, infrastructure, economies, and more. (The White House, 2021b)

The following identifies important perspectives on how climate change is recognized as a critical problem that can lead to disasters and to public health emergencies. Responses to these problems require extensive action by the federal government. An example of the need for government and private sector collaboration in addressing disasters and public health emergencies is the HHS Office of Climate Change and Health Equity (HHS, OCCHE, 2022), whose priorities are as follows:

- Identify communities with disproportionate exposures to climate hazards and vulnerable populations.
- Address health disparities exacerbated by climate impacts to enhance community health resilience.
- Promote and translate research on public health benefits of multi-sectoral climate actions.
- Assist with regulatory efforts to reduce greenhouse gas emissions and criteria air pollution throughout the health care sector, including participating suppliers and providers.
- Foster innovation in climate adaptation and resilience for disadvantaged communities and vulnerable populations.
- Provide expertise and coordinate to the White House, secretary of Health and Human Services and federal agencies related to climate change and health equity deliverables and activities, including executive order implementation and reporting on health adaptation actions under the United Nations Framework Convention on Climate Change.
- Promote training opportunities to build the climate and health workforce and empower communities.
- Explore opportunities to partner with the philanthropic and private sectors to support innovative programming to address disparities and health sector transformation.

All levels of government, nongovernmental organizations, and the private sector should be involved in implementing activities to meet the priorities in all types of communities, urban and rural.

Office of the Assistant Secretary for Health, U.S. Department of Health & Human Services, "About the Office of Climate Change and Health Equity (OCCHE)," 2022.

Examine the activities of the organization Health Care Without Harm. What is its purpose? Identify some of its activities. Consider how the activities relate to nursing and to public and community health. What impact might its activities have on disasters and public health emergencies?

Website: https://noharm.org/

Public Health Emergencies

"The Secretary of the Department of Health and Human Services (HHS) may, under section 319 of the Public Health Service (PHS) Act, determine that: a) a disease or disorder presents a public health emergency (PHE); or b) that a public health emergency, including significant outbreaks of infectious disease or bioterrorist attacks, otherwise exists. The declaration lasts for the duration of the emergency or 90 days, and may be extended by the Secretary. Congress must be notified of the declaration within 48 hours, and relevant agencies, including the Department of Homeland Security, Department of Justice, and Federal Bureau of Investigation, must be kept informed" (HHS, PHE, 2019). This represents the law or authority to make a critical decision that impacts many people.

COVID-19 is the most recent major public health emergency declared in the United States, and it is a communicable disease public health emergency. In May 2022, President Biden decided to renew the declaration for another 90 days. The law requires that states are given 60 days' notice of changes such as ending the declaration (CNN, 2022). Why was this decision made? The rate of infections is still high and increasing; however, the declaration has advantages for emergency management response and recovery. For example, the declaration makes it easier to provide free testing, therapeutic treatment, and vaccines for some populations, which will be eliminated when the declaration ends. The declaration makes it easier for Medicare to modify rules related to the use of telehealth, expanding use beyond rural areas for beneficiaries, and using this method for home visits. An important advantage is that "states are not involuntarily disenrolling residents from Medicaid during the declaration in exchange for receiving more generous federal matching funds. As many as 14 million people could lose Medicaid coverage after the emergency ends" (CNN, 2022).

There have been other epidemics, though none as major as COVID-19, such as Ebola, the Zika virus, and the H1N1 flu outbreak, which are communicable diseases. But some epidemics are not; for example, the current opioid crisis is viewed as a public health emergency. Weather-related events have also been designated as public health emergencies such as major hurricanes, floods, tornados, earthquakes, and fires as they impact public health and safety. Often weather-related disasters are not national but are focused on one or several states or locations in a state. Once an emergency is declared, public officials can make decisions and policies without going through the legislative process—speeding up the process to take actions. This might be referred as emergency powers to take certain actions, such as controlling freedom of movement, implementing evacuations, use of private property by emergency management, use of government resources, suspension of sale of alcohol, halting business, suspension of usual government business, deploying military personnel, and so on (Haffajee et al., 2014). The COVID-19 pandemic was declared a public health emergency and nationally communities experienced changes such as the closing of restaurants, changes in hours for business, changes in public transportation, and other requirements to protect the public's health. State government can also declare emergencies, and all states did this during the COVID-19 pandemic and have done this for other emergencies.

Public health emergencies may require the use of isolation and/or quarantine. **Isolation** is a term used in acute care when patients who have communicable diseases or at risk for them are kept separate and staff take certain precautions. However, it can have another meaning, which we heard a lot during the COVID-19 pandemic, when people were told to stay in their own homes and communities to prevent them from getting a communicable disease but had had no known exposure to the disease. **Quarantine** "separates and restricts the movement of people who were exposed to a contagious disease to see if they become sick" (HHS, CDC, 2017).

Government, Nonprofit and Humanitarian Organizations, and the Private Sector: Roles and Responsibilities

This section discusses the roles and responsibilities of government, humanitarian organizations, and the private sector in assisting communities as they prepare for disasters and public health emergencies and respond to these crises. Collaboration and coordination are important aspects that all stakeholders need to recognize as important.

Government: Local, State, Federal, and Global

The following describes the local, state, federal, and global levels of government responsibilities related to disasters and public health emergencies and how they interact to provide efficient and effective responses.

Local Government

Local government also has a major role and certain responsibilities in preparing for disasters and responding. Local government officials know their communities and its issues better than officials and can often do much more in encouraging public–private collaboration. Critical components of local government that need to be involved are law enforcement, fire department, infrastructure, emergency transport services that may be managed by government, social services, and even the school system. Local government also typically has relationships with faith-based organizations and nonprofit organizations in the community. Local government, whether a small town, city, or county need to coordinate with state government and others within the state. Local planning should be included in state planning, with special consideration given to budget and resources.

State

State governments are very involved in emergency management for disasters and public health emergencies. They are the frontline in planning prevention and preparedness as well as response. State governments know their populations, collect data that can be used in planning, know the major stakeholders, and should have good networking with local communities. They also serve as the key liaisons between local governments, the state government, and federal government. State governments should also have significant communication procedures and relevant policies to guide decisions and leadership during times of crisis.

Because of the Constitution there are some things the federal government cannot dictate to states. This means there is variation in how states might respond and even prepare. There are also political differences between states, which might lead to different decisions during times of crisis. Later in this discussion there is information about declaring public health emergencies; in this case the federal government may have influence over a state's decision. State governments have a public health mandate, and they have included public health services in their government organization. State public health services should network and collaborate with local public health services throughout the state. This includes planning for preparedness, collecting data, analyzing data, implementing when needed, sharing supplies and equipment, and developing the workforce.

Effective state disaster and public health emergency planning needs to include an effective statewide communication system and an effective evaluation process during recovery. All critical state departments need to be involved, for example law enforcement, fire and rescue, health care organizations, education at all levels, public transportation, the business community, funding sources, nonprofit and humanitarian organizations within the state, and all other organizations, departments, and agencies that might be required.

Federal

The CDC is the nation's health protection agency. It provides this protection by conducting research, collecting data such as surveillance and epidemiological statistics, and providing health information. Its major goals are as follows (HHS, CDC, 2022a):

- Detecting and responding to new and emerging health threats
- Tackling the biggest health problems causing death and disability for Americans
- Putting science and advanced technology into action to prevent disease
- Promoting healthy and safe behaviors, communities, and environments
- Developing leaders and training the public health workforce, including disease detectives
- Taking the health pulse of our nation

These goals relate to public health emergencies, with the CDC focused on developing public health leadership and resources at local, state, and national levels. The agency provides information and resources for emergency preparedness and response (HHS, CDC, 2022b).

In April 2022, the CDC announced the creation of a center for forecasting and outbreak analytics "to enhance the nation's ability to use data, models, and analytics to enable timely, effective decision-making in response to public health threats for CDC and its public health partners" (HHS, CDC, 2022c). The Center for Forecasting and Analytics (CFA) collaborates with local, state, and federal government levels based on the need to predict, inform, and innovate, applying information from COVID-19 to future public health emergencies. This should improve decision-making and responses. CFA is also collaborating with academic institutions and their experts to expand resources and evidence-based decisions. The center, as is true for current HHS activities and all its components, ensures that equity and accessibility are elements that are considered in its activities.

The HHS includes the Office of the Assistant Secretary for Preparedness and Response (ASPR), which focuses on medical and public health preparedness for response and recovery from disasters and public health emergencies. To accomplish this, ASPR "collaborates with hospitals, healthcare coalitions, biotech firms, community members, state, local, tribal and territorial governments, and other partners across the country to improve readiness and response capabilities" (HHS, ASPR, 2022a). Currently, ASPR is focused on responding to COVID-19, restoring decreased resources and a diminished workforce caused by the pandemic, and preparing for future emergencies. In the spring of 2022, ASPR started its process to develop the National Health Security Strategy (NHSS) for 2023–2026. A public request went out via the internet asking for stakeholders to respond to the following questions to provide information for the plan (HHS, ASPR, 2022b):

- What are the most critical national health security threats and public health and medical preparedness, response, and recovery challenges that warrant increased attention over the next five years?
- What medium-term and long-term (i.e., over next five years) actions should be taken to mitigate these challenges at the federal government and/or state, local, tribal, and territorial level?
- What public health and medical preparedness, response, and recovery opportunities or promising practices should be capitalized on over the next five years?

Nurses should respond to this type of call for comments and expertise to represent the nursing profession and its views of health care and practice and to advocate for patients, populations, and communities.

The Food and Drug Administration (FDA) is part of HHS and is responsible for protecting public health by "ensuring the safety, efficacy, and security of human and veterinary drugs, biological products, and medical devices; and by ensuring the safety of our nation's food supply, cosmetics, and products that emit radiation" (HHS, FDA, 2022). Some of its activities relate to disasters and public health emergencies. As we have seen with COVID-19, the FDA was critical in authorizing and approving testing methods and vaccines. It also dealt with misinformation that led to difficulties in ensuring public compliance. Some of its activities directly related to disasters are offering advice on use of medical devices in homes during disasters, consumer preparedness, information on food safety emergencies and alerts, and the National Disaster Call Center providing evacuation information. This may not be an agency that is thought of in coping with disasters and public emergencies, but drugs, medical devices, and food are critical aspects of a community and require attention during times of crisis. It may not always be easy to predict what might be a public health emergency. An example in 2022 is the national baby formula shortage. The FDA, as the federal agency that approves formulas, was involved in trying to resolve this problem, which led to concerns about meeting nutritional needs for babies and caused stress for families. Having expert guidance about prevention, preparing a response, responding, and addressing the aftereffects are important. In this public health emergency, the federal government applied the Defense Production Act to increase formula production quickly (Linton, 2022). The same law was used to increase production of COVID-19 vaccine and supplies needed for care of patients.

The National Institutes of Health (NIH), also part of HHS, is focused on research and seeking information to maintain and improve health, lengthen life, and decrease illness and disability (HHS, NIH, 2022). This research and examination of information not only focuses on basic science and acute care but also on public health needs and interventions. This guidance is used to prevent and prepare, respond, and evaluate actions during disasters and public health emergencies.

The overall mission of the Department of Homeland Security (DHS) is to protect the United States from threats, and one of these threats is disasters (DHS, Federal Emergency Management Agency [FEMA], 2022b). The DHS is part of HHS. FEMA is a DHS agency that focuses on disasters: assistance, response and recovery, resilience, and surge capacity force to provide more workforce to assist when FEMA cannot meet the needs, training, and technical assistance. FEMA's mission is to help people before, during, and after disasters. Its 2022–2026 strategic plan identifies the following goals for the agencies' activities (DHS, FEMA, 2022b):

1. Instill equity as a foundation of emergency management.
2. Lead whole of community in climate resilience.
3. Promote and sustain a ready FEMA and prepared nation.

FEMA has a national program and regional offices and a large budget. It employs many people, up to 20,000 nationwide, and this number increases during major disasters. The agency provides grants for pre- and post-emergency- or disaster-related projects, with some of the grants using a cost-share mechanism with the grantee. These grants may relate to the following (DHS, FEMA, 2022c):

- **Hazard mitigation:** Reducing or removing risk before a disaster such as planning, flood damage reduction, facility retrofitting, and forest or grassland fire management

- **Emergency food and shelter program:** Supplementing and expanding local nonprofit and governmental social services organizations that help reduce hunger and homeless (food, sheltering, supportive services)
- **Preparedness grants:** Nondisaster funds to support citizens and first responders (cybersecurity, public transportation systems, firefighters and law enforcement, training)
- **Resilience grants:** Dam safety, earthquake risk

To illustrate the impact of these grants, from January through March 2022, $7.9 million in grants were awarded to disaster survivors and 204 mitigation grants; 29 disaster declarations for states and counties; and 12 fire incident grants were awarded (DHS, FEMA, 2022c). One of the responsibilities of FEMA is to advise the president when a disaster declaration is under consideration. When local, tribal, or state government do not have the resources to effectively respond to a disaster government officials in this area may request that the president declare an emergency and then receive federal support. The president can declare a national emergency and a major disaster. FEMA assists in this decision-making process by assessing the situation and considering the extent of the disaster, the impact on individuals and public facilities, and the types of federal assistance that may be required and shares this assessment with leadership.

The HHS secretary can declare a public health emergency but would also consult with public health experts and with the president. The secretary needs to "determine that: a) a disease or disorder presents a public health emergency (PHE); or b) that a public health emergency, including significant outbreaks of infectious disease or bioterrorist attacks, otherwise exists" (HHS, ASPR, 2022c).

Global

World Health Organization (WHO, 2022), established in 1948, is "the United Nations agency that connects nations, partners and people to promote health, keep the world safe and serve the vulnerable—so everyone, everywhere can attain the highest level of health." One of its major goals is to direct and coordinate the world's response to health emergencies. For example, in the spring of 2022 the WHO was involved with the Afghanistan crisis (a health and humanitarian crisis, response to the COVID-19 epidemic within this country, need for medical supplies and health care services, trauma needs, etc.). Another example is the Northern Ethiopian humanitarian crisis due to conflict resulting in trauma and injuries; food insecurity and malnutrition; sexual- and gender-based violence; communicable diseases such as malaria and cholera; as well as reduced access to treatment for noncommunicable diseases and maternal and child health services. The Syrian crisis, which was an extended political and socioeconomic crisis resulting in severe deterioration of living conditions and an inadequate health system impacted by the COVID-19 pandemic. The Ukraine conflict with Russia is another global public health emergency that has led to stress on the Ukraine's health care system, with many deaths of civilians and military personnel, destruction of homes and entire communities, businesses, agriculture, and many people relocating to other countries. The WHO monitors or uses surveillance to assess disease outbreaks and has been the key global monitor of COVID-19. It is also involved in monitoring and responding to environmental emergencies such as floods and major storms.

The United Nations (UN, 2022a) is an international organization founded in 1945. Currently, it is made up of 193 member states and functions globally. The UN focuses on five major areas: (a) maintaining international peace and security, (b) protecting human rights, (c) delivering humanitarian aid, (d) supporting sustainable development, and (e) climate action; and it upholds international law. The organization has evolved internationally as needs change, but it continues to be an organization that engages many nations in working together, discussing common problems, and finding shared solutions that benefit all (UN, 2022b). Supporting the need for global attention to disasters and public health emergencies, the UN Office for Disaster Reduction (UNDRR, 2022) focuses on the UN system for the coordination of disaster reduction. An example of its activities is its START series, Skills and Technology Accelerating Rapid Transformation, which examines how cities could better prepare and mitigate disasters by improving disaster-preparation training.

It is predicted that there will be an increase in disasters by 2030. In 2015 there were 400 events per year, and by 2030 there is expected to be 560 per year (UNDRR, 2022). Extreme heat, which can cause droughts and then impact agriculture and food shortages, and can increase risks of large fires, is expected to be part of climate change problems. About 90% of disaster spending is for emergency relief, with only an estimated 4% spent on prevention and an estimated 6% on recovery. Not every major storm or hurricane results in major destruction and loss of life and is a financial drain on countries, but many are. Understanding risk and preparedness makes a difference on outcomes in emergency management, as does funding for preparedness, response, and recovery.

Nonprofit and Humanitarian Organizations

Nonprofit and humanitarian organizations have critical roles and responsibilities in disaster and public health emergency preparedness and response and may focus on one country or globally. Humanitarian organizations or NGOs assist people who are at risk and suffering, for example during armed conflicts, famines, and natural disasters. These organizations may be small or quite large, with many staff, volunteers, and funding, which is provided by donations and gifts. Though the government does provide some funding, these organizations are independent of government. They function locally, in states, at the national level, and globally. The following describes some examples of these organizations and their activities.

The International Federation of Red Cross (IFRC) and Red Crescent Societies is the world's largest humanitarian organization, involving 192 countries and over 14 million volunteers. IFRC notes in its 2022 strategic plan that much has been done to respond to COVID-19, but also there are other problems that need to be addressed, such as those associated with climate change, continuing concerns that may remain with COVID-19 and future communicable diseases, future health crises, disasters, and migration. Some of the IFRC (2022b) activities related to disasters are as follows:

- IFRC Go is the IFRC emergency operations platform for capturing, analyzing, and sharing real-time data during a crisis, allowing the IFRC network to better meet the needs of affected communities.
- The Disaster Response Emergency Fund (DREF) is the quickest, most efficient, and most transparent way of getting funding directly to local humanitarian authorities—both before and immediately after a crisis hits.
- Forecast-Based Action by the Disaster Response Emergency Fund (FbA by the DREF) is IFRC dedicated funding mechanism that helps National Red Cross societies take early action before disasters strike.

The International Committee of the Red Cross (ICRC), created in 1863, helps people globally during armed conflict, protecting victims. It remains neutral and active in addressing many problems such as sexual violence, migrants/refugee/asylum seekers' support and safety, health, mine action, water and habitat, and other problems that may occur in countries. The ICRC collaborates with the IFRC to protect and assist refugees and internally displaced persons (IDPs). Examples of activities are camp security, where refugees and IDPs may be living, mine clearance and awareness in locations where mines still exist, and providing training and guidance related to international humanitarian law and refugee law (UN, 2022c). The ICRC has also been very active in assisting countries with the COVID-19 pandemic. Nurses have long been a critical part of the Red Cross—as staff and volunteers across the globe provide care to refugees.

Another example of an NGO that focuses on the environment and climate change is the Global Facility for Disaster Reduction and Recovery (GFDRR). This organization, established in 2006, is a global partnership focusing on assisting countries that are low or middle income. The goal is to increase understanding of these countries' vulnerability and initiate interventions to better understand and reduce their vulnerability, particularly related to natural hazards and climate change. Funding for its work comes from multiple donors (GFDRR, 2022).

Other NGOs that may become important in providing services and support are faith-based organizations, academic institutions, and nonprofit organizations such as a local Red Cross and other similar organizations. They all should work together with government.

The Private Sector

Effective response to disasters and public health emergencies is dependent on government response and support, as described previously; however, the private sector must also participate. Understanding roles and responsibilities is important in developing effective collaboration, and this should be done prior to experiencing a disaster or public health emergency. After the experience, it is important to evaluate the process and outcomes and apply what is learned to prepare for future needs.

The first obvious area of the private sector that needs to be actively involved is the health care delivery system, which is often private and not governmental. Health care organizations, such as acute care hospitals, trauma centers, emergency services within hospitals or free-standing emergency clinics, emergency transport services that may be private, clinics, pharmacies, mental health, long-term care facilities, home health care agencies, and other health services are provided by the private sector. When these services and organizations are managed by the government they should be included in the planning, preparedness, and response. These services are dependent on infrastructure, some of which are part of the private sector. Examples of infrastructure that need to be effective or there needs to be alternative methods used to provide the services during a disaster are electricity, water, and a communication system.

Businesses also must consider planning for response to disasters, and they also need to prepare for public health emergencies. As we have seen with COVID-19, there has been a direct impact on businesses such as closing and reducing hours, working from home, wearing masks, and physical distancing. How did this change business activities and the issue of employee vaccine requirements and monitoring compliance? How did these factors impact customer/client relationships? Businesses were not prepared for this epidemic, but they may be better prepared in the future. Weather can also cause disasters that impact businesses, and this requires preparedness, particularly for businesses in areas that have a higher risk for this type of disaster such as tornados, blizzards or periods of extreme cold, and hurricanes.

> Developing resilient communities against all hazards requires leadership from government and business. Preparing the work-force, building safe facilities, investing in supplier relationships, and connecting to the community are all key pillars of true business community resilience—from the boardroom to the storefront. The path to leadership involves connecting with the right people and resources and committing to action by helping the business community and whole community mit-igate the hazards they face and bounce back quickly after an incident. Plus, it can decrease the overall costs of disruptions and disasters. (HHS, DHS, 2021a)

To accomplish this requires community business leaders to participate by connecting, integrating, coordinating, collaborating, committing, and sharing information. They need to ensure that their staff are prepared and can stay safe during a disaster; take steps to evaluate, mitigate, and reduce physical, cyber, and operational risks; ensure access to needed supplies and collaborate with supply resources; and work with community leaders, other businesses, emergency staff and planners, and elected officials in preparedness efforts and update as needed, and then participate in implementing plans when required.

There are other elements of a community that need to be considered as they have a direct impact on how people cope as well as their stress levels. Consider the following as examples of private-sector activities and their impact during a disaster or public health emergency:

- Access to money from the banks, for example inability to access funds through electronic means
- Limited access to grocery stores or stores unable to complete credit card transactions
- Grocery stores unable to get required deliveries when needed
- Refrigeration in grocery stores not functioning and not being able to safely store food
- Limited access to gas for automobiles
- Road closures that may limit personal travel, emergency travel for responders, stocking supplies, and moving equipment needed to respond to structural damage
- Electricity limited or not functioning, in the winter or in intense heat; cannot access heat or air conditioning, lack of refrigeration for home food

- Limited access for stores (grocery, hardware, pharmacies) to restock supplies so that the community and prepare, for example for a hurricane

There are many parts of the private sector that can have an impact or how a community responds to a disaster or public health emergency. Using effective preparedness that considers as many of these problems as possible should be part of effective public–private collaboration. Preparedness is discussed later in this guide.

Review the fact sheet on the Regional Disaster Health Response System (RDHRS) found at this link. What region do you live in? What other states included in your region? Review the accomplishments, and identify four accomplishments that that you think are important and require nursing input and leadership in communities.

Website: https://www.phe.gov/Preparedness/planning/RDHRS/Documents/RDHRS-Fact-Sheet-March2021-508.pdf

Emergency Management

Before beginning this section, see **Exhibit 1** to review some of critical terms related to disasters, public health emergencies, and emergency management.

Exhibit 1. Disaster and Public Health Emergency Terminology

Community Emergency Response Team (CERT): A community-level program administered by the FEMA; trains citizens to understand their responsibility in preparing for disaster, to safely help themselves, their family, and their neighbors. CERT volunteers provide immediate assistance to victims in their area, organize spontaneous volunteers who have not had training, and collect disaster intelligence to assist professional responders with prioritization and allocation of resources following a disaster.

Federal Emergency Management Agency (FEMA), "Glossary," https://training.fema.gov/programs/emischool/el361toolkit/glossary.htm.

Crisis Response Team: A team trained to assist in the healing process of students and staff following a traumatic event or incident.

Disaster: An occurrence of a natural catastrophe, technological accident, or human-caused event that has resulted in severe property damage, deaths, and/ or multiple injuries.

Drill: A type of *operations-based* exercise that is a coordinated, supervised activity usually employed to test a single, specific operation or function in a single agency.

Emergency management/response personnel: Includes federal, state, territorial, tribal, substate regional, and local governments, NGOs, private sector organizations; critical infrastructure owners and operators, and all other organizations and individuals who assume an emergency management role (emergency or first responder).

Evacuation: The organized, phased, and supervised withdrawal, dispersal, or removal of students, personnel, and visitors from dangerous or potentially dangerous areas.

Hazard: Something that is potentially dangerous or harmful, often the root cause of an unwanted outcome.

Hazard mitigation: Any action taken to reduce or eliminate the long-term risk to human life and property from hazards. The term is sometimes used in a stricter sense to mean cost-effective measures to reduce the potential for damage to a facility or facilities from a disaster or incident.

Incident: An occurrence, natural or human caused, that requires a response to protect life or property. Incidents can, for example, include major disasters, emergencies, terrorist attacks, terrorist threats, civil unrest, wildland and urban fires, floods, hazardous materials spills, nuclear accidents, aircraft accidents, earthquakes, hurricanes, tornadoes, tropical storms, tsunamis, war-related disasters, public health and medical emergencies, and other occurrences requiring an emergency response.

Incident action plan (IAP): A document outlining the control objectives, operational period objectives, and response strategy defined by incident command during response planning.

Incident command: The Incident Command System organizational element responsible for overall management of the incident and consisting of the incident commander (either a single or unified command structure) and any assigned supporting staff.

Jurisdiction: A range or sphere of authority. Public agencies have jurisdiction at an incident related to their legal responsibilities and authority. Jurisdictional authority at an incident can be political or geographical (e.g., federal, state, tribal, local boundary lines) or functional (e.g., law enforcement, public health, school).

Logistics: The process and procedure for providing resources and other services to support incident management.

Mass care: Actions taken to protect evacuees and other disaster victims from the effects of the disaster; providing temporary shelter, food, medical care, clothing, and other essential life support needs to the people who have been displaced because of a disaster or threatened disaster.

Mitigation: Includes activities to reduce the loss of life and property from natural and/or human-caused disasters by avoiding or lessening the impact of a disaster and providing value to the public by creating safer communities; to fix the cycle of disaster damage, reconstruction, and repeated damage. These activities or actions, in most cases, will have a long-term sustained effect; examples include structural changes to buildings, elevating utilities, and cutting vegetation to reduce wildland fires.

Natural hazard: Hazard related to weather patterns and/or physical characteristics of an area. Often occur repeatedly in the same geographical locations.

Preparedness: A continuous cycle of planning, organizing, training, equipping, exercising, evaluating, and taking corrective action in an effort to ensure effective coordination during incident response. Within the National Incident Management System (NIMS), preparedness focuses on the following elements: planning, procedures and protocols, training and exercises, personnel qualification and certification, and equipment certification. Examples include conducting drills, preparing homework packages to allow continuity of learning if school closures are necessary, and so on.

Prevention: Actions to avoid an incident or to intervene to stop an incident from occurring. Prevention involves actions to protect lives and property. Examples include cyberbullying prevention, pandemic influenza sanitation measures, building access control procedures, and security systems.

Public information: Processes, procedures, and systems for communicating timely, accurate, and accessible information on an incident's cause, size, and current situation.

Public information officer (PIO): A member of the command staff who serves as the conduit for information to internal and external stakeholders, including the media or other organizations seeking information directly from the incident or event.

Recovery: Encompasses both short- and long-term efforts for the rebuilding and revitalization of affected communities. Examples include short-term recovery focus on crisis counseling and restoration of lifelines, such as water and electric supply, and critical facilities. Long-term recovery includes more permanent rebuilding.

Recovery plan: A plan developed to restore an affected area or community.

Relocation: A common procedure implemented when the school building or environment surrounding is no longer safe. Students and staff are moved to an alternative facility where parents/guardians can reunite with children and/ or teaching can continue. Related words include parent–student reunification. During and following a disaster some residents may also need to relocate due to unavailable safe housing.

Resources: Personnel and major items of equipment, supplies, and facilities available or potentially available for assignment to incident operations. Resources are described by kind and type and may be used in operational support or supervisory capacities at an incident or at an emergency operations center.

Response: Activities that address the short-term, direct effects of an incident. Response includes immediate actions to save lives, protect property, and meet basic human needs and also includes the execution of emergency operations plans and mitigation activities to limit the loss of life, personal injury, property damage, and other unfavorable outcomes. Examples include lockdown, shelter-in-place orders, evacuation of students, search and rescue operations, and fire suppression.

Shelter in place: A common procedure implemented in the event of a chemical or radioactive release or time of violence. People take immediate shelter, sealing up windows and doors, and turning off air ducts or staying at home, school, or business sites until the all clear is announced.

Special needs population (vulnerable population): A population whose members may have additional needs before, during, and after an incident in functional areas, including but not limited to maintaining independence, communication, transportation, supervision, and medical care. Individuals in need of additional response assistance may include those who have disabilities, who are from diverse cultures, who have limited English proficiency, who are non-English speaking, or who are transportation disadvantaged.

Warning: The alerting of emergency response personnel and the public to the threat of extraordinary danger, for example, a hurricane or winter storm.

Watch: Indication by the National Weather Service that in a defined area, conditions are favorable for the specified type of severe weather such as flash floods, severe thunderstorms, tornadoes, and tropical storms.

Source: U.S. Department of Homeland Security, Federal Emergency Management Agency. (2022). *Glossary.* https://training.fema.gov/programs/emischool/el361toolkit/glossary.htm

Emergency Management Process: Phases

Emergency management is the organization and development of resources and the identification of roles and responsibilities needed to respond to a disaster or a public health emergency. It includes four phases: mitigation, preparedness, response, and recovery. The National Incident Management System (NIMS) is part of FEMA and guides government (local, state, national), nongovernmental, and private sectors and collaborates and coordinates with all necessary stakeholders on national, state, and local levels during the emergency management phases. See **Figure 1** describing the phases (DHS, 2016, p. v).

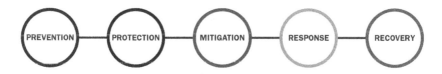

Figure 1.   Emergency management phases.

The following information provides a description of activities and examples related to the emergency management phases. Communities at the local, state, and federal level and even at the global level need to consider each of these phases as they develop preparedness plans to address disasters and public health emergencies. As we have experienced with COVID-19, planning and response to this public health emergency was not as effective as needed. Applying what has been learned from this experience to future incidents that will require emergency management is critical. We also need to recognize that there is increasing risk for natural disasters that require emergency management. What needs to be done in each of the phases?

Prevention

Prevention is the first emergency management phase. The activities in this phase focus on "the capabilities necessary to avoid, prevent, or stop a threatened or actual act of terrorism. Within the context of national preparedness, the term 'prevention' refers to preventing imminent threats" (HHS, DHS, 2016, p. v). The prevention phase includes consideration of disaster **frequency**; in other words, are there frequent types of disasters that might occur in one area, for example a state in which there are large numbers of tornadoes during certain times of the year? Predictability is also an important aspect of understanding prevention of disasters and emergency public health. Some disasters have a higher level of predictability than others, for example a hurricane. We know that certain areas of the country are at risk for hurricanes during certain times of the year and hurricanes can be tracked before they impact land. However, bioterrorism is a less predictable risk and yet it is a critical risk event. Prevention considers the types of disasters that might occur and the hazards within a community and then attempts to develop interventions to lower the risk. This does not guarantee that there will be no disasters or public health emergencies. For example, interventions to reduce the risk of communicable diseases are important, such as use of masks and physical distancing, but one can still be exposed. Interventions may be taken if there are chemical hazards due to industrial processes in a community, ensuring that safety procedures are followed and alerts are activated when there is a problem. Areas with high fire risk need careful assessment to reduce risk. These areas often have fire watch efforts, especially during the high seasons of fire risk and use methods to reduce brush, provide campers with information about care of cooking fires, be alert during electrical storms, and other interventions. In areas of high risk for flooding steps need to be taken to prevent excessive water in certain areas, repair dams and ensure that bridges are secure, and that business and residential areas near the flood zones are protected. Security is another intervention that is used to prevent violence, such as such as security at airports or in schools. Though this does not guarantee there will not be incidents of violence or a terrorist attack, it does reduce the risk. Prevention takes time and planning and must be ongoing. Interventions need to be evaluated to determine if they are still effective as preventative measures.

Protection

The **protection** phase focuses on "the capabilities necessary to secure the homeland/country against acts of terrorism and manmade or natural disasters" (DHS, 2016, p. v). Examples of common protection measures are evacuation, sheltering, sheltering in place, lockdowns, masking and physical distancing, isolation, and quarantine. Evacuation is concerned with getting out of a house or building; ideally there should be two exits and stairwells, and elevators should be used with care, and in some situations elevators should not be used. Evacuation may also involve people moving from a location, typically quickly to avoid harm. Sheltering requires getting to a protected area, for example when there is a tornado warning getting into a covered area, basement, and so on, may be for a short term or longer requiring overnights. To shelter in place means to get to a safe area and stay there until the alert is removed. This is the type of alert that we hear more now during times of violence in communities and schools. Lockdowns are also used during times of violence. The term was common during the COVID-19 pandemic in some communities and countries when people were told not to leave their homes except for food shopping and medical needs.

Mitigation

Mitigation focuses on activities used to reduce loss of life and property by lessening the impact of disasters or public health emergency (DHS, 2016, p. v). It requires an understanding of risk and resilience, recognizing that disasters cannot always be avoided. Reducing loss of life and property decreases the negative impact of a disaster and may assist in gaining strength to deal with future disasters. When prevention and mitigation are compared, mitigation focuses on reducing the severity to the people involved in the disaster and to the community whereas in prevention interventions are used to reduce the risk of even having a disaster or a public health emergency. Mitigation typically occurs before disaster or public health emergency. The same is true for prevention. Mitigation and prevention are closely related and should be considered together when communities begin to plan and prepare for disasters and public health emergencies.

Some examples of mitigation measures that might be taken by a community include ensuring effective use of building codes, mapping out flood areas; encouraging residents to prepare tornado-safe rooms, particularly in states that have a high frequency of tornadoes; burying electrical cables in high-risk areas for low temperatures during the winter months; hazard mapping, or understanding the risk of hazards in the community and applying this information; ensuring communities have effective insurance plans available to them for the risks they might experience; and providing public education programs in advance of a disaster to prepare residents for possible responses and to encourage the use of preventative measures.

Healthy People 2030 (see **Appendix B**) includes an objective to increase the proportion of people who have an emergency plan for disasters (HHS, ODPHP, 2022d). The fact that Healthy People includes this topic in its objectives indicates that this is an important public health issue. The disaster may vary, but preparation is important at all levels, including at the individual and family level.

Response

The **response** phase focuses on "capabilities necessary to save lives, protect property and the environment, and meet basic human needs after an incident has occurred" (HHS, DHS, 2016, p. v). This phase includes emphasis on actions taken by the emergency teams in the community, which may include volunteers, to respond to the actual disaster or public health emergency and to reduce the risk of mortality and morbidity. Disaster **triage** refers to identifying and then separating individuals who need more intensive care quickly. This requires training prior to a disaster as well as immediate access to victims. The site for triage can vary widely depending on the disaster or the public health emergency, for example flooding near water areas and fires can be variable as to their needs of the victims as well as supplies needed and access to victims. A triage system must be designed and included in the planning for disasters. Most emergency rooms have a triage procedure that is used, but in this case, we are talking about triage at the site of a disaster and then victims can be taken to health care facilities. This requires transportation and staff, and this too must be included in the planning. The number of casualties is a critical factor in determining the needs for the response team and supplies and transportation of those who were injured. This too is highly variable. In addition, time is an issue; for example, the recent collapse of an apartment building in Florida required time to search for victims. The victims were not found all at the same time, and many of them were not found alive. This requires additional services for those who do not survive.

It is critical to understand that there is no perfect scenario to describe a disaster or a public health emergency. There are too many variables that can be different, but there are some basics. An effective triage system is required to respond to those who have been injured with effective teams to communicate to one another. The healthcare system needs an emergency workforce, medical supplies, equipment, blood supplies, transportation, and very effective communication. In addition to the injured, there are other issues related to caring for those who are experiencing the disaster or the public health emergency. Some examples include food and water supplies, housing, personal items such as clothing, and so on. Information is also very important to those who are experiencing the disaster and should be part of the response. Emotional support is critical at this point, and often volunteers provide this type of support as well as local faith-based organizations. Response is complex. Nurses are very involved in these efforts either as part of the official emergency management team or as volunteers in their community. Student nurses may serve as volunteers during these times to help their community. It is important to assess the needs of people who have been involved in the disaster or the public health emergency and then institute interventions to respond to immediate needs. This does not mean that there will not be long-term needs during recovery; however, the foundation for recovery comes with the immediate response. The emergency management team needs to listen to those who are experiencing the disaster and try to respond to their needs as they arise. This may mean that the emergency management team needs to ask for additional help; for example, a local emergency management team may ask its state for help, or a state may ask for federal assistance.

Recovery

The **recovery** phase focuses on "the capabilities necessary to assist communities affected by an incident to recover effectively" (HHS, DHS, 2016, p. v). This phase, as is true for all the other phases, is also complex and highly dependent on the type or disaster or public emergency the community has experienced. The types of populations in the community and their needs prior to the incident are also important; these needs do not go away, and they may be much more complex after the disaster. For example, if the community has a high level of older adults with complex or chronic health problems, after the disaster they may need more support services. If a community's health care system has been damaged by the disaster or the public health emergency, this too will be a critical factor in the recovery phase. For example, during the height of COVID-19, many hospitals experienced staff shortages and had staff leave. They are now dealing with this problem after a major communicable disease experience.

Recovery requires intensive assessment of needs of all parts of the community, which includes residential areas and their residents, businesses, financial systems such as the banks, school systems, transportation, the local or state government, and infrastructure. After this assessment, repair takes place, and this may be long-term depending on the destruction or the needs of the community. Funding is critical during this phase and must be considered for all components of the community. Further information is provided in this guide on relief during these times. In addition, it becomes very important to collaborate and communicate with many organizations and groups in a community, as they will provide much of the support needed for individuals and families; nearby communities may also assist. The school system is an important aspect of recovery. If it has been affected by the disaster or the public health emergency, the education system will need to review its needs and funding for changes that might be required. Basically, the whole community needs to be assessed to determine needs, to eliminate those areas that require no changes or additional support, and then to focus on what needs to be repaired or improved. Recovery takes time, and this can be quite stressful for members of the community who want things back where they were before the incident occurred.

Emergency Management Structure

In 2022, the CDC developed a public health capability framework to assist jurisdictional public health agencies in designing their structure to ensure effective preparedness—supporting the CDC's center for Public Health Emergency Preparedness (PHEP)—and established cooperation among many agencies in the United States. There have been revisions made in this framework based on evaluations and identified needs. The current focus areas or domains are community resilience, incident management, information management, countermeasures and mitigation, surge management, and biosurveillance. The following are the focus areas for the most current standards (HHS, CDC, 2019):

- Community preparedness
- Community recovery
- Emergency operations coordination
- Emergency public information and warning
- Fatality management
- Information sharing
- Triage
- Mass casualty care
- Medical countermeasure dispensing and administration
- Medical material management and distribution
- Medical surge
- Nonpharmaceutical interventions
- Public health laboratory testing
- Public health surveillance and epidemiological investigation
- Responder safety and health
- Volunteer management

Preparedness

Preparedness, as defined in Exhibit 1, is the "continuous cycle of planning, organizing, training, equipping, exercising, evaluating, and taking corrective action in an effort to ensure effective coordination during incident response" (DHS, FEMA, 2022).

The federal government provides tools and resources for communities to use in emergency management. It is the key resource for all stakeholders who are involved in emergency management and preparedness Examples of some of these tools and resources are as follows:

- The Healthcare and Public Health (HPH) Risk Identification and Site Criticality (RISC) toolkit is an objective, data-driven all-hazards risk assessment that is designed to be used by public and private organizations that are part of the HPH to assist in emergency preparedness planning, risk-management activities, and resource investments. This provides standards-based evaluation criteria that can be accessed and used with directions to ensure easy application (HHS, ASPR, 2021).

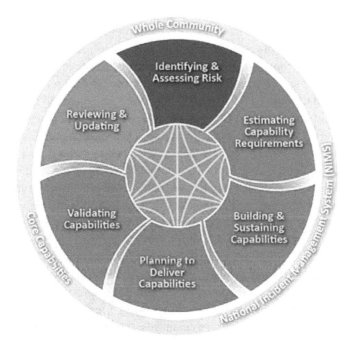

Figure 2. Components of the National Preparedness System.

- The HHS emPOWER Program is a partnership between the Office of the Assistant Secretary for Preparedness and Response (ASPR) and the Centers for Medicare and Medicaid Services (CMS). This program provides federal data, mapping, artificial intelligence tools, and training and resources to help communities nationwide, with a focus on protecting the health of at-risk Medicare beneficiaries. This population includes 4.4 million individuals who live independently and rely on electricity-dependent durable medical and assistive equipment and devices and essential health care services. Public health authorities and their partners in all 50 states, five territories, and the District of Columbia use emPOWER program data and tools to strengthen emergency preparedness, response, recovery, and mitigation and take action to protect at-risk populations (Medicare and Medicaid beneficiaries) prior to, during, and after incidents, emergencies, and disasters (HHS, ASPR, 2022d).

Communities (local, state, and national) need to identify where they will locate the **Emergency Operations Center** (EOC) and determine the type of facility that will be used. This center directs operations during an event;

given the nature of the event it may be temporary, but some communities may have a more permanent site that may be operationalized as need. Typically, the local fire, law enforcement, and health care services in which the incident occurs are the most involved in organizing and maintaining the EOC. Access to past and current data is an important part of the activities so that decision-making can be efficient and effective. Data collection is important both for current functions but also necessary for evaluation post-recovery and preparing for future disasters and public health emergencies.

Developing an emergency management plan begins with a risk assessment to identify potential emergency incidents. For example, if a community is prone to hurricanes, this would be one of the possible types of disasters. All government segments, businesses, health care organizations, schools, and so on should develop a plan that considers its employees, clients/customers/students/patients, visitors, contactors, and anyone who might be involved with the organization or facility. The plan must recognize that the first concern is safety for any incident, which is an occurrence, natural or human caused, that requires a response to protect life or property. This means preparing for emergency first aid, extinguishing fires, use of fire drills and evacuation, recognizing danger of chemicals, threat or presence of explosive materials and actions to take, protection of building damage and areas to use for greater protection such as a basement, and back-up plans for loss of electricity and water.

Emergency management uses a structure to support the process and meet all the needs of each of the phases. The Incident Command System (ICS) is the organizational element responsible for overall management of an incident and includes the incident commander and any assigned supporting staff. The **incident action plan** (IAP) describes the control objectives, operational period objectives, and response strategy defined by incident command during response planning. Emergency management/response personnel are associated with federal, state, territorial, tribal, substate regional, and local governments; NGOs; private sector organizations; critical infrastructure owners and operators; and all other organizations and individuals who assume an emergency management role (emergency or first responder). To be effective drills or operations-based exercises, coordinated, supervised activities are usually used to test a single, specific operation or function in a single agency to ensure the team is prepared.

Other resources that may be used are the **Community Emergency Response Team** (CERT). This is a community-level program administered by the FEMA that trains citizens to understand their responsibility in preparing for disaster and to safely help themselves, their family, and their neighbors. CERT volunteers also provide immediate assistance to victims in their area. As needs may change quickly, they may organize additional volunteers who have not had the training. They also collect disaster data to assist professional responders with prioritization and allocation of resources following a disaster—assisting in ongoing assessment. The **Crisis Response Team** (CRT) includes trained members who assist in the healing process in an organization, business, community, or population (neighborhood, school, and so on) following a traumatic event or incident. This resource is typically used after a violent incident such as a school shooting or violence in a business location. This is part of the response phase but extends into recovery.

Emergency management staff, or **first responders**, are associated with all levels of government, nongovernmental organizations, private sector organizations (businesses, financial), social services, infrastructure (e.g., water and electrical utilities, fire department, law enforcement), and health care services and sites. They are the key people who implement a preparedness plan and follow it through all the emergency management phases.

Emergency medical services (EMS) must be assessed and included in preparedness. This assessment should address personnel (needs and number, competencies, locations, access, and any regulatory issues), facilities EMS will use, required supplies and equipment, and transportation for personnel and those needing assistance and care. Emergency management must also consider the needs of EMS such as food and water for staff and volunteers, rest areas and personal needs, ability to communicate with their families, and so on.

It is necessary to plan logistics, the process and procedure for providing resources and other services to support incident management. This must consider transportation methods and staff, such as drivers and people to move supplies, food and water, and equipment; may require special transfer equipment; gas; and status of the local roads and highways. In some situations, planes may be used to bring in supplies, equipment, and staff, so this must be considered as plans are made. In addition, in some disasters a community may ask for help from nonaffected areas, for example for electrical repairs, and this requires support services for the workers who come in, such as temporary housing, food, water, and so on.

Assessment of needs is part of preparedness, and it is a complex area as the needs range from preexisting medical problems, minor injuries, trauma and intensive care, and death, which requires plans for handling of the deceased, identification, may require autopsy and care of bodies, and contact of family members and others who need to know mortality data. Consideration needs to be given to factors such as schools, long-term care facilities, ages of the population, institutions such as mental health, serving people with disabilities, prisons or jails, typical use of home health care, and so on. Diverse populations need to be identified, particularly when developing public communication to ensure that language is considered. This assessment requires sharing of information and coordination with all levels of the health care system.

Identifying possible health care specialty care needs is part of emergency management, along with identifying how these needs will be met. Are medical specialists available, and if not, how might they be accessed, for example, from another location? What are the medical supplies and equipment that might be required, and how does the community access them?

An ongoing plan (emergency operations plan) is needed to ensure all who work in emergency management know how people and property will be protected; it should also identify clear roles and responsibilities; describe communication process and policies and procedures; identify required personnel, supplies, and equipment; and describe clear structure and reporting.

Collaboration, Coordination, Communication

Collaboration and coordination are critical ongoing activities throughout the emergency management process. Federal, state, local, tribal, and territorial emergency response stakeholders must be involved and work with all aspects of the community to ensure needs are identified and met. In general, public health agencies are directly involved during disasters and public health emergencies and are key members of the emergency management preparedness process. They work with other health care services to ensure a broad range of health services are available. Health needs that were important prior to an incident continue to be important, though during some disasters or public health emergencies prior health needs may go unmet or other methods may need to be used to receive health care. For example, greater use of telehealth reduces the need for patients to go into clinical sites and allows them to get advice for their problems. As is true with any adjustments, there must be consideration given to barriers that may limit use of alternative methods. Telehealth requires connection to Wi-Fi and devices, and if these are not available, this method will not be effective and may make it worse as people will be frustrated. In addition, this may highlight equity issues, with some areas having limited funds for devices, not having electricity, and so on.

Communication is a critical element of emergency management. The staff and volunteers must be able to communicate effectively and quickly. However, communication with the public is also critical. Public health emergencies require sharing clear information so that people understand their risk and know what steps they can take to protect themselves (WHO, 2017). Risk communication and involves experts, community leaders, government officials, and the people who are at risk—providing real-time accurate information. The United States, and all countries, have struggled with communicating with the public during the COVID-19 pandemic. We were not prepared for this, and many mistakes were made. The big challenge is there are many communication methods, and many of them are out of the control of authorities and experts. The internet makes this possible. It can be used to communicate effectively, but the lack of control makes this difficult. Some communities and countries use apps that citizens have on their mobile phones and other devices to alert citizens quickly, share information, and so on. This can be helpful. Social media, however, provides a way for many people to share opinions and incorrect information. Misinformation, incorrect or misleading information, is not helpful, increases stress and distrust, and can lead to poor decisions. This is a critical public health communication issue for emergency management and preparedness and must be monitored in all the emergency management phases. Collaboration, coordination, and communication require that those helping a community recognize challenges before they become challenges and try to resolve them to get services needed at the time needed in the places needed to meet the essential public health services (see **Appendix A**).

In 2020, the National Advisory Council report to the FEMA administrator addressed three important questions (DHS, FEMA, 2020):

1. What should be the future vision of emergency management and FEMA in 2045? How should FEMA and its nonfederal partners address an outlook of increasing disasters and downward pressure on federal funding?
2. Given the downward federal budget pressures and upward natural hazard trends, what are the best ways to build capacity in response, recovery, preparedness, and mitigation at the local, tribal, territorial, and state levels?
3. What actions should FEMA take to ensure marginalized and vulnerable communities can recover quickly? How can FEMA better structure its programs to meet the needs of the most vulnerable populations, especially women and children?

The report's recommendations were that FEMA should focus on equity, outcomes, coordination, and on effectiveness, applying the guiding principles of equity, resilience, efficiency, professionalism, accountability, and science-based, data-driven, and collective processes. The report noted that FEMA programs are not serving those who most need them, and financial assistance often is not always equitable. An example is FEMA uses property ownership as a key factor in initiating damage assessments, leaving out people who rent and the homeless. This approach provides more financing to wealthier areas of a community that have been damaged by a disaster.

Another potential barrier is access to FEMA staff and information for assistance, which is often done through technology, and some segments of a community may not have this access even before the disaster. Even use of a mobile phone or any telephone may be difficult if communication systems are down. The report emphasizes that the goal in providing resources and support should be to people with the greatest needs. It is important that emergency management develop trust in all segments of the community to improve preparedness. Communities that are resilient and have high social capital have a greater ability to respond and recover from disasters and public health emergencies. Social capital refers to networks, relationships in the community that support the functions of the community—living and working in the community. All should work to ensure efficient and effective collaboration, coordination, and communication for positive outcomes.

Do you know your community's plan for a natural disaster? How might you find out about it? Are nurses mentioned in the plan? If so, what information is shared on the nursing roles and responsibilities? What is your school's plan for a disaster response?

Experiencing Disasters and Public Health Emergencies

"Disasters, natural and technological, profoundly affect the health and well-being of communities, especially those in disaster-prone regions. ... Vulnerable communities face cumulative, not isolated, threats, and disparities [that] exacerbate the impact of each overlaying risk domain. ... Protecting the most vulnerable is the proven strategy to protect all" (Lichtveld, 2018, p. 28). Many communities have not supported vulnerable populations during times of disasters by not developing effective preparedness that considers their usual status, equity, and impact of disparities. Communities may provide limited support in recovery (funding, resources) and not recognize the stress that some people in the community experience routinely due to disparities, and then the community neglects to factor in the stress of a disaster or a public health emergency, which exacerbates the level of stress. It is important to approach disaster recovery as a long-term process. Communities with less resilience going into a disaster will have a longer, harder recovery. Chronic community stressors will continue to be a problem. "Disaster aid must prioritize those most vulnerable, regardless of race, ethnicity, income, and citizen status. One potentially daring but promising strategy is to elevate community resilience as an essential public health service and consequently integrate community resilience measures as performance benchmarks of federal, state, and local health agencies" (Lichtveld, 2018, p. 30). See **Appendix A** to review the current public health essential services.

Vulnerable Populations

"At-risk individuals are people with access and functional needs that may interfere with their ability to access or receive medical care before, during, or after a disaster or emergency" (HHS, CDC, 2017). There are many types of vulnerable populations. Vulnerable populations that are of particular concern during a disaster or public health emergency are children and older adults; people with chronic illnesses and disabilities; people who may not be able to live independently or need some support; people who have limited or no transportation access, which impacts actions such as evacuation; people who need regular access to medical care; people with communication problems; and populations that regularly experience socioeconomic problems. The CDC recognizes the important need to include planning to assist vulnerable populations in emergency preparedness. To support this view, the CDC notes the following (HHS, CDC, 2017):

- Seventy-one percent of the people who died during Hurricane Katrina were older than 60.
- There is an 80% chance that a person will experience a temporary or permanent disability in their lifetime.
- Twelve percent of the U.S. population, ages 16–64, have a special health care need due to disability.

Many people are at greater risk during a disaster or public health emergency.

A vulnerable population that may be ignored in emergency management planning is people residing in long-term care facilities, which may have several levels of services and care based on needs of residents. These organizations should have their own preparedness and should also be integrated into their community's preparedness. The residents of these facilities have complex needs, and mobility of residents is often compromised. Another related group are people in the community who are receiving home health care and may need electricity for medical equipment or are receiving complex care such as oxygen in the home, which requires support and equipment. This is not always an older population, as others have homecare health needs. It is important that home healthcare agencies develop plans and engage in community planning. Homecare agency staff need to help their patients and families with their personal preparedness—using many of the government resources to guide them along with guidance from the agency plan.

Review the following sources of examples for personal preparedness. How might you apply this information as a home health care nurse in your community to a patient and family?

Websites: https://www.ready.gov/plan
https://www.fema.gov/press-release/20210318/how-build-kit-emergencies
https://www.cdc.gov/cpr/infographics/pfe-family.htm

Due to concern about social vulnerability the CDC developed a minority health social vulnerability index (SVI; HHS, CDC, OMH, 2021). The SVI is used to assess health equity in research, planning, designing programs and responses, and evaluating responses to disasters and public health emergencies. The factors included in the assessment index are socioeconomic status, household composition and disability, minority status and language, housing type and transportation, healthcare infrastructure and access, and medical vulnerability. This type of tool is useful when a community wants to have a better understanding of the needs of all its residents.

Responses to Disasters and Public Health Emergencies

Community health resilience (CHR) is "the ability of a community to use its assets to strengthen public health and healthcare systems and to improve the community's physical, behavioral, and social health to withstand, adapt to, and recover from adversity" (HHS, ASPR, 2015). How does a community develop resilience? HHS recommends the following strategies:

- Strengthen and promote access to public health, health care, and social services.
- Promote health and wellness alongside disaster preparedness.
- Expand communication and collaboration.
- Engage individuals who may be at risk and programs that serve them.
- Build social connectedness.

Nurses who work in public and community health should have an awareness of the community's resilience and understand how this applies to specific populations and neighborhoods.

Disaster Relief

The federal government is involved in disaster relief activities. The Robert T. Stafford Disaster Relief and Emergency Assistance Act, PL 100-707, 1988, amended the Disaster Relief Act of 1974, PL 93-288, is the legislative authority for most federal disaster response activities, especially FEMA and FEMA programs. The law supports funding to local and state governments to assist in disaster-relief activities. The law also gives the president the power to declare a national emergency and to make funds available to respond to the emergency or major disaster. Before the president can declare an emergency, the governor(s) of the involved states must determine that the state cannot handle the emergency and lacks sufficient resources, usually after using the available state resources. There is then communication between the governor(s) and the president. The law provides for three types of assistance (FindLaw, 2022):

- **Individual assistance:** Assistance directly given to individuals and businesses affected by an emergency/disaster
- **Public assistance:** Funding and expertise allocated to state and local governments
- **Hazard mitigation assistance:** Funding aimed at eliminating or reducing the long-term effects of the disaster

The question of the use of quarantine may come up, particularly for public health emergencies. This law "does not explicitly give the president the ability to quarantine citizens at a time of disaster. Rather, the federal government, in times of health emergencies, may have the power to quarantine citizens under the commerce clause of the Constitution" (FindLaw, 2022). The HHS (2022b) and CDC are involved in this type of decision, including isolation, by providing data, analysis, and expertise.

Recovering from a disaster is a gradual process and many require assistance during an incident or in recovery. Disaster assistance or **relief** is "financial or direct assistance to individuals, families and businesses whose property has been damaged or destroyed and whose losses are not covered by insurance" (IIIIS, DHS, 2021b). This assistance or relief covers expenses that cannot be covered in other ways. Examples of assistance to individuals are rental assistance, lodging expense reimbursement, home repair assistance, and home replacement assistance. Other types of housing-related expenses may be covered, such as personal property assistance, transportation, and moving and storage assistance. In some situations, assistance may be provided for funerals, medical and dental services, and childcare. Businesses also may receive assistance. This assistance is critical in reducing stress and allowing people to move forward and deal with problems during recovery.

Nongovernmental and humanitarian organizations are also involved in providing relief, such as the American Red Cross, which may be active during and after a disaster. It may provide emergency financial assistance immediately after a disaster, long-term assistance for individuals and families, and grants to communities. The organization gets most of its funds from donations and notes that a greater portion of donations go to services rather than to maintain the organization's administration (American Red Cross, 2022).

Urban and Rural Areas

Urban areas are complex and are places where large numbers of people reside, go to school, and work. Infrastructure is complex as it is designed to meet many needs of the population, which is often very diverse and with a high population density. Living in urban areas requires access to public transportation, typically several type; social services to meet needs of a diverse population; healthcare services to meet broad age groups; employment opportunities; and access to food stopping and other needs. Urban local government has a high level of responsibilities to meet the diverse needs of its citizens. Urban areas also have diverse living situations, such as rentals (apartment and single-family houses), housing ownership (apartments and single-family houses), shared housing, and homelessness, in addition to community members living in supportive facilities such as long-term care. Each type of housing requires some variation in needs during a disaster. For example, mobilizing resources and experience is a critical activity and involves all levels of government down to local government and officials. Urban areas have similar needs as rural areas during incidents, but they may be organized differently and have greater budgets, staff, equipment, supplies, and other resources than rural areas and must provide services to a larger population.

In 2021, the WHO recognized the importance of improving urban preparedness in an extensive report. The WHO (2021) framework focuses on the following:

- Governance and financing for health emergency preparedness
- Multisectoral coordination for preparedness
- High population density and movement
- Community engagement and risk and crisis communication
- Groups at risk of vulnerability
- Data, evidence, and information
- Commerce, industry, and businesses
- Organization and delivery of health and other essential services

Figure 3 provides an overview of preparedness in cities and urban areas.

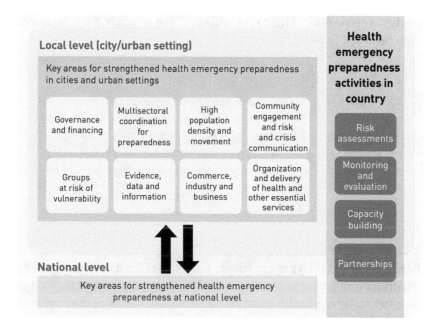

Figure 3. Strengthening overall health emergency preparedness—the role of cities and urban settings.

Rural areas also have unique characteristics that impact their needs and responses during disasters or public health emergencies. A critical factor in these areas is that they often have insufficient health providers and services prior to a disaster or public health emergency—physicians, including specialists, nurses and other healthcare professionals, labs, acute care, emergency care, pharmacies, home health care, and long-term care. Then, when they are hit with a community-wide emergency, they struggle to meet additional needs. The economic status of the community is often weak, with people struggling in agriculture, finding employment, and dealing with costs of living and health care. In addition, they may have less income from taxes, which impacts community services and staffing.

People frequently travel long distances. However, many of these communities have social connectedness, strong faith-based institutions, and active citizens. These strengths need to be used during times of emergencies. They often need more relief if a disaster causes major destruction to homes, businesses, government services, social services, utilities, and transportation such as roads. Rural areas need clear plans to prepare for these times. Often these areas experience common, frequent disasters, often weather-related such as wildfires, floods, droughts, tornados, and other storms. Some prediction is possible if they have a history, and typically these incidents occur in certain seasons.

After reviewing the information on urban and rural settings, consider how each type of setting impacts public health nursing during a disaster or public health emergency. With your student team, or independently, identify at least four urban and four rural characteristics, their impact how an urban or rural area might differ in problems during and after a disaster, and how this might impact nursing response and services.

Stress and Trauma

Resilience is the ability to experience and recover from a disaster. It is an important component of the national effort to prepare for and respond to disasters and public health emergencies so that communities can cope with and recover from these incidents. What can be done to strengthen communities so that when that when these incidents occur they can better cope with the experience and recover more quickly? This is a key question related to preparedness, and it is also a question that relates to how individuals, families, populations, and communities feel about their experience—during and after the incident. It is important to understand that many factors can impact resilience. SDOH have an impact, for example if a community has socioeconomic problems prior to a tornado that then causes destruction to homes, businesses, and infrastructure, it is harder for people to cope during the incident and to recover. Public health emergencies are also impacted by the status of the community due to their health status, age, and diversity. This was seen with COVID-19 when older adults had more serious problems if they had COVID-19 or if people had other prior medical problems such as respiratory, cardiac, or immune suppression health problems. This all weakens individuals' resilience, and it also has an impact on population and community resilience as more health care and other services will be required and may not be available at the level required during a disaster or public health emergency and in recovery.

Individual resilience impacts community resilience and vice versa. All need to take actions to reduce risks. Being resilient and prepared have a positive impact on outcomes. Individual households need to engage in preparedness, just as local communities, states, and the national level must do to maintain community resilience. All require clear communication and understanding of the communication process during disasters and public health emergencies.

This understanding must be part of planning and shared before an incident. People should not struggle to find information during an incident, and they should know how to get reliable information quickly. Communities need to routinely assess the status of preparedness of individual households, businesses, and other organizations in the community and their level of understanding of how to respond to an incident and access information.

Cumulative community vulnerability occurs when communities experience frequent disasters and are disaster-prone, such as due to climate. These communities confront stressors and often do not fully recover before another disaster occurs; an example is a hurricane area. Recovery is related to individuals, families, and communities but also to infrastructure and public health services. Litchveld (2018) recommends adding elevating community resilience to the essential public health services. Though this has not been officially done, it is recognition that it is important in public health in general and not just during a disaster or public health emergency (see **Appendix A**).

Community members with a history of mental health problems often find it difficult to cope with added stress during a disaster or a public health emergency. Most people experience stress, anxiety, depression, and other responses but may have better coping skills than people with prior coping problems. Reactions may occur in any age group and at any point during the incident or after it. Taking care of self is important. Children need clear information, and support and, when possible, they need to continue their usual routine. If they cannot go to school, this is an additional stressor. Health care workers and responders need to be very aware of the impact of stress and assess individuals, families, populations, and communities for signs of ineffective coping. Some of these signs are as follows (HHS, CDC, 2018):

- Feelings of fear, anger, sadness, worry, numbness, or frustration
- Changes in appetite, energy, and activity levels
- Difficulty concentrating and making decisions
- Difficulty sleeping or nightmares
- Physical reactions such as headaches, body pains, stomach problems, and skin rashes
- Worsening of chronic health problems
- Increased use of alcohol, tobacco, or other drugs

Stress can also affect personal relationships with family and friends. The development of marital problems, as well as acting-out behavior in children, is not uncommon. Ineffective problem solving may interfere with making wise decisions such as what to do about housing, financial problems, and other issues related to recovery. This problem may even extend to difficulty completing daily routines. Asking for help may be easy for some people but not for others. This means screening and identifying people who may be at risk and may be demonstrating these feelings, reactions, and behaviors is important, and then providing support or treatment as needed.

Some victims and responders may experience **posttraumatic stress disorder** (PTSD), which can be a long-term and more serious response. PTSD may result in reliving the event (flashback, nightmares), avoidance of situations that relate to the event, and increased arousal such as sleep problems, irritability, and violence. Some people with PTSD may experience depression, panic attacks, and suicidality. This is a serious medical problem that requires treatment.

Movement of Populations: Refugees, Displaced Persons

Disasters and public health emergencies of all kinds may result in the need to assist refugees and displaced persons. However, some types of disasters tend to increase the risk of people becoming refugees, such as war and conflict. **Refugees** are persons who cross borders from one country to another due to fear for their safety. This has been experienced in the last years in the Middle East and Africa, with refugees fleeing to Europe. This movement of people may save lives, but it also has a major impact on the refugees and the countries they move to for safety. They are traumatized, come with little personal belongings and money, often do not know the language, and may have limited job skills. All ages are involved, and many come with health problems. In most situations the new country is unprepared for the sudden influx of refugees, who require all types of needs: housing, clothing, food, health and social services, transportation, education, employment, and so on. In most cases, the refugees will not return to their home country, so the burden on the new country is long-term and complex. There are also political issues that arise and issues of acceptance and discrimination.

Displaced persons are people who must move within their own country due to a disaster or public health emergency, a move that may be temporary and experienced multiple times or permanent. A common example is weather-related disasters such as hurricanes, floods, fires due to drought, and so on. Displaced persons have complex needs, but typically at some point they will return to their homes after recovery, though this may take a while to accomplish.

The most recent example of refugees and displaced persons is the war in Ukraine, which now has brought an estimated 12 million people, mostly women, children, and the elderly, to many European countries. This refugee group suddenly found themselves running for their lives, often leaving behind husbands and fathers and other adult male family members, and leaving with few personal items. Many in this group are babies and children, and they will carry this experience with them for the rest of their lives. This is a tremendous burden for these countries. In addition, an estimated 7 million are displaced within Ukraine, often moving from place to place or living in shelters. Most have lost their homes permanently or experienced major damage to their homes and communities, schools, and businesses. With many civilians and military dying or injured, the people are also experiencing loss of family members and others, with little opportunity to grieve in a manner they would during peaceful times

Displaced persons can be a problem during a disaster when people need to evacuate to safety, often for short periods of time, for example during a hurricane some people may need to go to another city or state for shelter. Disaster preparedness should include plans for providing shelter and other needs for displaced persons until they can return to their homes. It is a burden to care for displaced persons—it takes staff, funds, the use of services that might otherwise be used by the local permanent population, housing, and so on. This may lead to community stress and complaints, especially after the initial phase of "we will help those who need." As the time passes, reevaluation is needed to ensure that not only the needs of displaced persons are met but that the continuing needs of local community members are considered. The rush to volunteer and donate time, money, and supplies is not endless, especially as recovery progresses. Housing needs may change over time as people need to move from communal shelters to group housing, and to individual housing units. Employment and financial support also changes over time.

Impact on the Future

Part of the emergency management process is planning for future needs: Is there risk that there will be other disasters of similar type or public health emergency or other types? What can be learned about planning and response that can be applied to other possible future incidents? Emergency management needs to include extensive evaluation of its preparedness plans, implementation in all phases, and its outcomes. This requires feedback from all stakeholders and data. This information should then form the basis for review and revisions of preparedness and be applied to future needs. Communities at all levels should periodically review their preparedness plans and the make adjustments as needed; for example, consider changes in population characteristics and needs, resources, funding, and research that can be used to improve and provide evidence-based strategies. This is not a plan that should be filed away and then pulled out at the time of a disaster or public health emergency. Nurses should be involved in all phases of this process and recognize that planning for future incidents and needs is long-term.

Nursing Roles and Interventions in Disasters and Public Health Emergencies and Crisis Response

Nurses who work in all areas of health care have the potential of being involved in disasters and public health emergencies. Disaster nursing has been described as "doing the most, for the least, by the fewest" (Veenema, 2013, p. 231). Nurses have responsibilities related to incidents (disasters and public health emergencies) that can occur in any community. These nursing roles and responsibilities depend on where nurses typically practice or where they might practice during an incident. It is important that nursing education prepare students for disasters, public health emergencies, and crisis responses. The following content discusses these issues and roles and responsibilities in disaster and public health emergency: practice, education, management, consultation, advocacy, and research (ICN, 2017).

The Nursing Profession's View of Disasters and Public Health Emergencies

The nursing profession has been engaged in leading nurses to assume active roles in disasters and public health emergencies. Nursing organizations are involved and have included this critical concern in health care delivery in their policies and recommendations. The American Academy of Nursing has issued statements about climate change and health, advocating that "nurses play essential roles in public health, clinical care, emergency services, research, and advocacy through their work to reduce and respond to the health consequences of climate change" (Leffers & Butterfield, 2018, p. 210). The academy recommends the following related to policies that should be considered (Leffers & Butterfield, 2018):

1. Reduce sources of pollution that contribute to climate change.
2. Assure and fund robust systems for climate change monitoring and public health tracking.

3. Educate the public so that they understand the connections between their health and climate health.
4. Advance training initiatives that improve nurses' ability to implement sustainability initiatives in healthcare systems.
5. Urge the American Colleges of Nursing (AACN) and HRSA to develop curricula and professional development opportunities to increase the knowledge and skills of the healthcare workforce to effectively address the health impacts of climate change.
6. Urge the American Nurses Association to incorporate climate change and health into the *Scope and Standards of Practice: Nursing* to require effective response into clinical practice for the care of persons affected by climate change.
7. Collaborate with governmental and nongovernmental organizations addressing emergency responses to climate change-related disasters. (pp. 211–212)

The ANA (2020) recognizes the importance of disasters and public health emergencies in its 2020–2030 strategic plan. Enhancing nurses' disaster preparedness capabilities is included in its goal to evolve the practice of nursing to transform health and health care.

The Future of Nursing™ Campaign for Action includes the need to prepare nurses for disasters and public health emergencies in its recommendations, noting that this activity should also address inequities (Future of Nursing™ Campaign for Action, 2021). Nurses should collaborate with nursing organizations, health care organizations and insurance, nonprofit organizations, federal government, and other organizations such as businesses. Nurses are a critical stakeholder in all the emergency management phases. The campaign identifies the need for the CDC to establish a National Center for Disaster Nursing and Public Health Emergency Response. The relevant federal government departments and agencies, such as HHS, CDC, AHRQ, CMS, HRSA, and ASPR, should address issues related to professional regulation (licensure), funding for preparation and training, and so on. Key nursing organizations (ANA, NLN, etc.) need to support and increase licensure examination content related to disaster and public health emergency content and nursing responsibilities. Health care employers also need to expand and clarify nursing roles during these events and make greater use of nursing expertise. All of these recommendations indicate that nurses are important in providing efficient and effective health care during disasters and public health emergencies.

Nursing research in disaster and public health emergencies is as important as it is in other areas of health care. A review of 247 studies related to this overall topic concluded that common focus areas for these studies are mental health outcomes and psychosocial well-being, preparation and planning for deployment in disasters, and training (Hugelius, 2021). Areas that have had limited examination are assessment, intervention, recovery, safety and security, incident management systems, and law and ethics. This indicates there are topics that need more nursing research so that nurses can continue to lead and practice effectively during disasters and public health emergencies.

Public and Community Health Nursing in Disasters and Public Health Emergencies

Nurses need to be engaged in all the steps of emergency preparedness. The ANA (2015) *Code for Nurses with Interpretive Statements* includes content that relates to this need and discusses this concern in the ANA 2017 issue brief: "Who Will Be There? Ethics, the Law, and a Nurse's Duty to Respond to a Disaster." The brief covers many factors related to nurses but makes the point that nurses provide care during these events and at the same time must care for themselves, which includes their families. This may cause a conflict of obligation and ethics. This type of incident puts nurses at risk, as we learned from the COVID-19 pandemic, but also occurs with other types of disasters and public health emergencies such as climate-related events.

Generally, the public views nurses positively and trusts them, and this can assist nurses as they work with the public during times of crises. Public health nurses have many skills that are important in preparing and responding to these incidents such as an emphasis on the community and populations, team-based care, a holistic approach to health care, knowledge of the community, advocacy, and consideration of health equity and SDOH. Nurses have expertise that can make a difference in health care services such as knowledge of health and psychological responses, communication skills, knowledge of population health and communities, understanding of planning and implementation of plans, ability to work with diverse teams (interprofessional, consumers, government, humanitarian organizations within the community, etc.), knowledge of the health care system and how it functions, and the ability to provide education to the public. The nursing process (assessment, diagnosis, planning, intervention, evaluation) is applied in the emergency management phases. Nurses have responsibilities related to risk reduction, response and recovery planning and interventions, and providing care. They need to work to support resiliency and ensure equity and access to not only health services but also social services, which requires them to work with social service staff in planning and response. Nurses recognize that community members need not only services for physical responses and problems but also those for mental health, which requires psychosocial support for all ages experiencing a disaster or public health emergency. Providing psychological first aid (PFA), which is "a set of skills that helps community residents care for their families, friends, neighbors, and themselves by providing basic psychological support in the aftermath of traumatic events," is an important intervention during all emergency management phases (HHS, CDC, 2019).

Nurses typically, even when there is no disaster, coordinate and collaborate with a variety of community services, such as emergency services, emergency transportation and response, fire departments, law enforcement, long-term care settings, senior centers, home health care agencies, schools, and local government. Nurses should serve on planning committees and task forces to ensure effective preparedness and advocate for their community needs. They are excellent resources to provide public education on preparedness in a variety of settings such as community centers, schools, community activities such as fairs, within health care settings, and so on. Examples of specific roles and responsibilities for nurses related to disasters and public emergencies are as follows:

- Leadership and planning
- Community assessment
- Contact tracing
- Screening
- Providing nursing care (mass care center, triage, emergency department, intensive care)
- Consumer education (individuals, families, populations)
- Surveillance
- Infection control
- Immunizations
- Mental health and crisis response
- Evaluation

To ensure that nurses provide these services, communities need nurses during times of disasters and public health emergencies. The workforce issue is complex; nurses have responsibilities that are not directly connected to these incidents, as they provide care routinely in hospitals and public and community health. These events increase the need. In some situations, nurses from other states have moved temporarily to assist where there is need and shortage. Travel nurse agencies have assisted in providing additional nurses. In some cases, states have asked other states for help. A barrier or challenge is licensure. Registered nurse licensure is state based, so one cannot just go practice in another state if not licensed in that state. In the last few years, a change that was made to assist more rapid transition to practice in some states is the Nurse Licensure Compact (NLC):

> With multistate licensure, nurses from multiple states were easily able to respond and supply vital services in other NLC states. Primary care nurses, nurse case managers, transport nurses, school home health and hospice nurses, among many others, needed to routinely cross state boundaries to provide the public with access to nursing services, especially in states heavily impacted by the pandemic. Multistate licensure facilitated this process. (National Council of State Boards of Nursing [NCSBN], 2022a)

Multistate or compact licensure is not available in all states, but when states agree, typically neighboring states, nurses can practice in their home state and in states agreed on in their licensure state's compact relationship. This can help resolve emergency workforce needs, and it also provides nurses with more employment flexibility. In some situations, nurses may volunteer to provide public health services such as immunizations and care in shelters. These relationships between states require legislation, and this takes time to arrange.

Other sources for nurses are inactive and retired nurses. When workforce needs increased to a critical point during COVID-19, some states developed methods to allow these nurses to return to practice quickly. This is an example of how, during a time of crisis, innovation is required to ensure the health and safety of the public. In addition, some states reduced their requirement to have an active license in their states and accepted active licensure from other states for temporary practice during the pandemic and the extreme staff shortage and high hospitalization rates. The NCSBN concludes from the COVID-19 experience, "The spread of COVID-19 has shown that a virus is not impacted by boundaries. Neither should barriers to licensure. Now and in the near future, medical professionals across the country will seek to go where they are needed to provide vital care, by crossing state lines physically or via telehealth. While emergency declarations have temporarily lifted some restrictions on licensure, a crisis like the one we are facing is a sobering reminder that having all U.S. states and territories in the NLC would streamline this process for the next health crisis or natural disaster" (2020). It is important to recognize that the NCSBN cannot dictate to state boards of nursing as the boards of nursing are part of a state's government. The NCSBN (2022b) is "an independent, not-for-profit organization through which nursing regulatory bodies act and counsel together on matters of common interest and concern affecting public health, safety and welfare, including the development of nursing licensure examinations."

In 2022, the American Organization of Nurse Leaders (AONL) partici-pated in the Nurse Staffing Think Tank (American Association of Critical Care Nurses, 2022). The American Association of Critical Care Nurses and other nursing organizations such as the ANA participated in addressing staffing problems that have been exacerbated by COVID-19. We know that determining staffing levels is never easy, but during a disaster or public health emergency this becomes more complex with the need to meet routine health needs and emergency health needs, which may be impacted by residents relocating and changing needs. The task force identified several priority areas that need urgent action (American Association of Critical Care Nurses, 2022):

- Healthy work environment
- Diversity, equity, and inclusion
- Work schedule flexibility
- Stress injury continuum
- Innovative care delivery models
- Total compensation

Nurse leaders add expertise to preparedness teams. The following are examples of how nurse leaders augment teams with their ability to collaborate with others, problem-solve and assist others with this process, understand team leadership and effective team membership, collaborate with diverse groups, use effective communication with staff and consumers, understand healthcare finance, and ability to manage. Nurse leaders typically are effective crisis leaders.

Review the recommendations from the Nurse Staffing Task Force at the link pro-vided. It is clear the public health emergency (COVID-19) had a strong influence on the development of this task force and its work—though staffing was a prob-lem prior to this crisis. What is missing from the recommendations? Consider their primary focus.

Website: https://www.nursingworld.org/~49940b/globalassets/practiceand-policy/nurse-staffing/nurse-staffing-think-tank-recommendation.pdf

Another area that often is not considered is the political response in assuming an active advocacy role for individuals, families, populations, and communities. An example of advocacy is involvement in public policy devel-opment related to climate change, which is the greatest public health threat (Nicholas et al., 2020). The International Council of Nursing (ICN) supports the WHO's view on the dangers of climate change (ICN, 2021). Some of the disaster incidents that impact health are heat waves or any radical change in temperature, droughts, storms, floods, and rising sea levels. These changes increase risk of heat stroke, hypothermia and death and impact preexisting conditions such as cardiovascular, respiratory, and kidney problems. Floods can lead to traumatic injuries and death and the spread of vector- and water-borne infections. Nutrition may be compromised if agriculture is damaged or delayed. The latter can be due to human-caused disasters such as wars; for example, the war in Ukraine has delayed planting, damaged crops, and limited the transport of crops. Many countries depend on wheat from this area. **Figure 4** highlights the CDC's view on climate change and human health.

Advocacy supports the three public health core functions (see **Appendix A**) and prevention. Working to reduce climate change means health care providers such as nurses need to communicate with policymakers and government officials and collaborate to improve the environment. In addition, nurses are aware of the needs of vulnerable populations and the issue of health equity to reduce disparities. These populations and the impact of SDOH mean that some people experience more barriers during times of disasters, such as those related to climate change. These factors need to be discussed with policymakers.

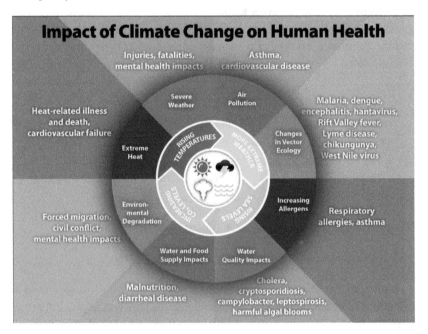

Figure 4.   Impact of climate change on human health.

The ANA is involved in advocating for improvement in preparedness and response to disasters and public health emergencies. In 2017 the organization published an extensive statement on nurses and their roles and responsibilities: "Who Will Be There? Ethics, the Law, and a Nurse's Duty to Respond to a Disaster". See link to review this statement. What is your opinion of the statement? Does it surprise you that a key nursing profession organization would discuss this topic in this detail? Discuss with your student team to hear what others have to say about this information.

Website: https://www.nursingworld.org/~4af058/globalassets/docs/ana/eth-ics/who-will-be-there_disaster-preparedness_2017.pdf

Nursing Education to Meet Health Care Needs for Disasters and Public Health Emergencies

Nursing education standards include emphasis on health equity, SDOH, population health, public health, and other related topics and clinical experiences in the community (AACN, 2021; NLN, 2022). The emphasis in this guide is on public and community health; however, when communities experience a disaster or a public health emergency all aspects of the health care system should be involved in planning, initiating actions, and evaluating for improvement. Nursing education needs to recognize that students should be guided to understand the entire health care system and need for a planned, effective responses. Some students may be in their nursing program when a disaster or public health emergency occurs. COVID-19 is one of those examples, as students had to cope with the responses to the pandemic while in clinical or adjust to changes in clinical and to distance education. Some students may experience natural disasters in their local communities, such as a major flood, and become involved in assisting during the response as part of clinical experiences or volunteering. Students and faculty should be aware of their school's and their community's plans for disasters and public health emergencies. Schools should also ensure that students are aware of plans that their clinical sites have developed for disasters and public health emergencies. Content that is important is epidemiology, infection control, immunizations, emergency care and trauma, psychological support and response, rapid assessment (of individuals, populations, and communities), health care worker responder safety, and communicating with the public.

One of the chapters in *The Future of Nursing 2020–2030: Charting a Path to Achieving Health Equity* discusses disaster preparedness and public health emergency response (NAM, 2021a). (See **Appendix C** for information about other NAM reports.) The emphasis in this chapter of the report is on nursing and what it has to offer in these situations. The report notes that there are concerns about the level of nursing education content. In examining nurse preparation in this area the report notes that 78% of the nurses surveyed had limited familiarity with emergency preparedness and disaster response (NAM, 2021a, 2021b). The report recommends actions to support nurses and their practice in disaster and public health emergencies:

- The CDC should establish a Center for Disaster Nursing and Public Health Nursing Response to improve nursing emergency preparedness.
- More support should be provided by federal agencies to prepare the nursing workforce related to nursing emergency preparedness.
- Nursing education programs and employers need to develop or expand disaster preparedness educational and training opportunities for all positions and settings.

These types of recommendations are policy related and connected to responses that need to be taken at the federal level and then impact state and local levels. All of them recognize that nurses have important roles and responsibilities, but they need to be prepared. An example of recommendations from other nursing organizations that agree with this report's recommendations are the ICN's (2019) disaster nursing core competencies (2nd ed.) and include the following eight focus areas:

1. Preparation and Planning
2. Communication
3. Incident Management Systems
4. Safety and Security
5. Assessment
6. Interventions
7. Recovery
8. Law and Ethics (p. 9)

Summary

This content examined the complex area of disasters and public emergencies. Emergency management addresses how communities respond to these incidents. Nurses are active in all levels, local, state, and federal, as well as global. They participate in activities during the phases of prevention, protection, mitigation, response, and recovery. Communities need to be prepared prior to a disaster or public emergency, and apply what they learn from previous incidents to their planning. The federal government is very active in preparedness, response, and relief, providing many resources that communities, health care professionals and other responders, and citizens can use to reduce risks and recover. Equity is of critical concern for all types of health care services, including disaster and public emergencies, and as we have learned from the COVID-19 pandemic, the most recent public health emergency, and some of the recent weather-related disasters, there can be serious disparities in how people receive services and in the types of services they receive negatively impacting outcomes. Attention needs to be given to equity, SDOH, and reducing disparities.

Discussion Questions

1. Why would a local disaster preparedness task force include nurses in the community on the task force? What types of nurses should be included?
2. Describe how you might prepare your home and family for a disaster in your community.
3. Compare and contrast refugees and displaced persons.
4. Why is it important to provide psychological support to individuals, families, populations, and communities during and after a disaster or a public health emergency?

References

American Association of Colleges of Nursing. (2021). *The essentials: core competencies for professional nursing education.* https://www.aacnnursing.org/Portals/42/AcademicNursing/pdf/Essentials-2021.pdf

American Association of Critical Care Nurses. (2022). *National nurse staffing think tank launched by leading healthcare organizations develops solutions tool kit to address staffing crisis.* https://www.aacn.org/newsroom/national-nurse-staffing-think-tank-launched-by-leading-health-care-organizations

American Nurses Association. (2015). *Code for nurses with interpretive statements.* Author.

American Nurses Association. (2017). *Who will be there? Ethics, the law, and a nurse's duty to respond to a disaster.* https://www.nursingworld.org/~4ad845/globalassets/docs/ana/who-will-be-there_disaster-preparedness_2017.pdf

American Nurses Association. (2020). *2020–2030 strategic plan*. https://www.nursingworld.
org/ana-enterprise/about-us/anae-strategic-plan-2020---2023/

American Red Cross. (2022). *Disaster relief*. https://www.redcross.org/about-us/our-work/
disaster-relief.html

Centers for Disease Control and Prevention Center for Preparedness and Response.
(2017). *Emergency preparedness & populations: Planning for those most at risk*. https://
stacks.cdc.gov/view/cdc/84021

Choi-Schagrin, W. (2021). More than 40 nations pledge to cut emissions from their
health industries. *The New York Times*. https://www.nytimes.com/2021/11/08/climate/
emissions-climate-change.html

CNN. (2022, May 17). *The Biden administration is continuing the COVID-19 public health
emergency declaration beyond July 15*. https://edition.cnn.com/2022/05/17/politics/
covid-19-public-health-emergency/index.html

FindLaw. (2022). *The Stafford Act explained*. https://www.findlaw.com/consumer/insurance/
the-stafford-act-explained.html

Future of Nursing™ Campaign for Action. (2021). *The National Academy of Medicine's
future of nursing 2020–2030 charting a path to achieve health equity: Recommendations
at a glance*. https://campaignforaction.org/wp-content/uploads/2021/07/Recommen-
dations-at-a-glance-5-21-21.pdf

Global Facility for Disaster Reduction and Recovery. (2022). *About us*. https://www.gfdrr.
org/en/feature-story/about-us

Haffajee, R., Parmet, W., & Mello, M. (2014). What is a public health emergency? *New
England Journal of Medicine, 371*, 986–988.

Hugelius, K. (2021). Disaster nursing research: A scoping review of the nature, content, and
trends in studies published 2011–2020. *International Emergency Nursing, 59*, 101–107.

International Council of Nursing. (2017). *Disaster nursing. International classification
for nursing practice (ICNP®) catalogue*. https://www.icn.ch/what-we-do/projects/
ehealth-icnptm/icnp-download/icnp-download

International Council of Nursing. (2019). *Core competencies in disaster nursing, version 2.0*.
https://www.icn.ch/sites/default/files/inline-files/ICN_Disaster-Comp-Report_WEB.
pdf

International Council of Nursing. (2021, October 11). ICN joins global health community's call for climate action ahead of COP26 to avert the "biggest health threat facing
humanity." https://www.icn.ch/news/icn-joins-global-health-communitys-call-climate-
action-ahead-cop26-avert-biggest-health-threat

International Federation of Red Cross and Red Crescent Societies. (2022a). *What is a
disaster?* https://www.ifrc.org/what-disaster

International Federation of Red Cross and Red Crescent Societies. (2022b). *Global plan
2022*. https://www.ifrc.org/global-plan-2022

Leffer, J., & Butterfield, D. (2018). Nurses play essential roles in reducing health problems
due to climate change. *Nursing Outlook, 66*, 210–213.

Linton, C. (2022). *Baby formula shortage: Biden to invoke Defense Production Act*. CBS News. https://www.cbsnews.com/news/baby-formula-shortage-biden-to-invoke-defense-production-act/

Litchveld, M. (2018). Disasters through the lens of disparities: Elevate community resilience as an essential public health service. *American Journal of Public Health, 108*(1), 28–30.

National Academy of Medicine. (2020). *Evidence-based practice for public health emergency preparedness and response*. National Academies Press.

National Academy of Medicine. (2021a). *Report brief: Nurses in disaster preparedness and public health emergency response*. https://nap.nationalacademies.org/resource/25982/FON%20One%20Pagers%20Disasters%20and%20Public%20Health%20Emergencies.pdf

National Academy of Medicine. (2021b). *The Future of Nursing 2020–2030: Charting a path to achieving health equity*. National Academies Press.

National Council of State Boards of Nursing. (2022a, February 28). *National Licensure Compact Commission annual report now available*. https://www.ncsbn.org/16648.htm

National Council of State Boards of Nursing. (2022b). *Home page*. https://www.ncsbn.org/index.htm

National League for Nursing. (2022). Nursing education competencies. https://www.nln.org/education/nursing-education-competencies

Nicholas, P., Gona, C., Evans, L, & Reid, E. (2021). The intersection of climate change and health: An explication of the Future of Nursing 2020–2030: Charting a path to achieve health equity. *Witness: The Canadian Journal of Critical Nursing Discourse, 3*(2). https://witness.journals.yorku.ca/index.php/default/article/view/114

Nelson, H. (2021). *Health equity necessary for public health disaster preparedness*. https://patientengagementhit.com/news/health-equity-necessary-for-public-health-disaster-preparedness

Raker, E., Arcaya, M. C., Lowe, S. R., Zacher, M., Rhodes, J., & Waters, M. C. (2020). Mitigating health disparities after national disasters: Lessons from the RISK project. *Health Affairs, 39*(12). https://www.healthaffairs.org/doi/10.1377/hlthaff.2020.01161

Robert Wood Johnson Foundation. (2021). *Climate change threatens our health and deepens health inequities*. https://www.rwjf.org/en/library/research/2021/09/climate-change-threatens-our-health-and-deepens-health-inequities.html

Robichaux, C., & Sauerland, J. (2021). The social determinants of health, COVID-19, and structural competence. *OJIN: The Online Journal of Issues in Nursing, 26*(2). https://ojin.nursingworld.org/MainMenuCategories/ANAMarketplace/ANAPeriodicals/OJIN/TableofContents/Vol-26-2021/No2-May-2021/Articles-Previous-Topics/The-Social-Determinants-of-Health-COVID-19-and-Structural-Competence.html

The White House. (2021a). *Executive order on tackling the climate crisis at home and abroad*. https://www.whitehouse.gov/briefing-room/presidential-actions/2021/01/27/executive-order-on-tackling-the-climate-crisis-at-home-and-abroad/

The White House. (2021b). *National Climate Task Force.* https://www.whitehouse.gov/climate/

United Nations. (2022a). *About us.* https://www.un.org/en/about-us

United Nations. (2022b). *Our work.* https://www.un.org/en/our-work

United Nations. (2022c). *What is a refugee?* https://www.unhcr.org/what-is-a-refugee.html

United Nations Office for Disaster Risk Reduction. (2022). *Home page.* https://www.undrr.org/

U.S. Department of Health and Human Services. (2022a). *Topic collection: Disaster and healthcare disparities.* https://asprtracie.hhs.gov/technical-resources/156/disasters-and-healthcare-disparity/0

U.S. Department of Health and Human Services. (2022b). *Who has the authority to enforce isolation and quarantine because of a communicable disease?* https://www.hhs.gov/answers/public-health-and-safety/who-has-the-authority-to-enforce-isolation-and-quarantine/index.html

U.S. Department of Health and Human Services, Centers for Disease Control. (2018). *Coping with a disaster or a traumatic event.* https://emergency.cdc.gov/coping/pdf/Coping_with_Disaster.pdf

U.S. Department of Health and Human Services, Centers for Disease Control and Prevention. (2019). *Public health emergency preparedness and response capabilities.* https://www.cdc.gov/cpr/readiness/00_docs/CDC_PreparednesResponseCapabilities_October2018_Final_508.pdf

U.S. Department of Health and Human Services, Centers for Disease Control and Prevention. (2022a). *Mission, role, and pledge.* https://www.cdc.gov/about/organization/mission.htm

U.S. Department of Health and Human Services, Centers for Disease Control and Prevention. (2022b). *Emergency preparedness and response.* https://emergency.cdc.gov/

U.S. Department of Health and Human Services, Centers for Disease Control and Prevention. (2022c). *CDC launches new center for forecasting and outbreak analytics.* https://www.cdc.gov/media/releases/2022/p0419-forecasting-center.html

U.S. Department of Health and Human Services, Centers for Disease Control and Prevention Center for Preparedness and Response. (2017). *Emergency preparedness & populations: Planning for those most at risk.* https://stacks.cdc.gov/view/cdc/84021

U.S. Department of Health and Human Services, Centers for Disease Control and Prevention, Office of Minority Health. (2021). *Minority health social vulnerability index fact sheet.* https://www.minorityhealth.hhs.gov/Assets/PDF/MH%20SVI%20Fact%20Sheet_7.15.2021.pdf?utm_medium=email&utm_source=govdelivery

U.S. Department of Health and Human Services, National Institutes of Health. (2022). *Mission and goals.* https://www.nih.gov/about-nih/what-we-do/mission-goals

U.S. Department of Health and Human Services, Office of Assistant Secretary for Preparedness and Response. (2015). *Community resilience.* https://www.phe.gov/Preparedness/planning/abc/Pages/community-resilience.aspx

U.S. Department of Health and Human Services, Office of Assistant Secretary for Preparedness and Response. (2021). *HPH Risk Identification and Site Criticality (RISC) toolkit 1.0.* https://www.phe.gov/Preparedness/planning/RISC/Pages/default.aspx

U.S. Department of Health and Human Services, Office of Climate Change and Health Equity. (2022). *About the Office of Climate Change and Health Equity.* https://www.hhs.gov/ash/ocche/about/index.html

U.S. Department of Health and Human Services, Office of Disease Prevention and Health Promotion. (2022a). *Social determinants of health.* https://health.gov/healthypeople/objectives-and-data/social-determinants-health

U.S. Department of Health and Human Services, Office of Disease Prevention and Health Promotion. (2022b). *Environmental quality.* https://www.healthypeople.gov/2020/leading-health-indicators/2020-lhi-topics/Environmental-Quality?source=govdelivery&utm_medium=email&utm_source=govdelivery

U.S. Department of Health and Human Services, Office of Disease Prevention and Health Promotion. (2022c). *Environmental health.* https://health.gov/healthypeople/objectives-and-data/browse-objectives/environmental-health

U.S. Department of Health and Human Services, Office of Disease Prevention and Health Promotion (ODPHP). (2022d). Healthy People 2030. https://health.gov/healthypeople/objectives-and-data/social-determinants-health

U.S. Department of Health and Human Services, Office of the Assistant Secretary for Preparedness and Response. (2022a). *About ASPR.* https://aspr.hhs.gov/AboutASPR/Pages/default.aspx

U.S. Department of Health and Human Services, Office of the Assistant Secretary for Preparedness and Response. (2022b). *Inform the development of the 2023–2026 national health security strategy.* https://aspr.hhs.gov/ResponseOperations/legal/NHSS/Pages/nhss-development-2023-2026.aspx

U.S. Department of Health and Human Services, Office of the Assistant Secretary for Preparedness and Response. (2022c). *Public health emergency declarations.* https://www.phe.gov/emergency/news/healthactions/phe/Pages/default.aspx

U.S. Department of Health and Human Services, Office of the Assistant Secretary for Preparedness and Response. (2022d). *HHS empower program.* https://empowerprogram.hhs.gov/

U.S. Department of Health and Human Services, Public Health Emergency. (2019). *Public health emergency declaration.* https://www.phe.gov/Preparedness/legal/Pages/phedeclaration.aspx

U.S. Department of Homeland Security. (2016). *National prevention framework.* https://www.fema.gov/sites/default/files/2020-04/National_Prevention_Framework2nd-june2016.pdf

U.S. Department of Homeland Security. (2021a). *Natural disasters.* https://www.dhs.gov/natural-disasters

U.S. Department of Homeland Security. (2021b). *Disaster assistance.* https://www.dhs.gov/disaster-assistance

U.S. Department of Homeland Security, Federal Emergency Management Agency. (2020). *National Advisory Council report to the FEMA administrator: November 2020.* https://www.fema.gov/sites/default/files/documents/fema_nac-report_11-2020.pdf

U.S. Department of Homeland Security, Federal Emergency Management Agency. (2022a). *Office of Equal Rights.* https://www.fema.gov/about/offices/equal-rights

U.S. Department of Homeland Security, Federal Emergency Management Agency. (2022b). About us. https://www.fema.gov/about

U.S. Department of Homeland Security, Federal Emergency Management Agency. (2022c). FEMA grants. https://www.fema.gov/grants

U.S. Environmental Protection Agency. (2022). *Health aspects of exposure to lead in drinking water.* https://www.cbsnews.com/news/flint-water-crisis-settlement-judge-approves-626-million/

U.S. Food and Drug Administration. (2022a). *What we do.* https://www.fda.gov/about-fda/what-we-do

Veenema, T. (2013). *Disaster nursing and emergency preparedness for chemical, biological, radiological, and terrorism and other hazards.* (3rd ed.). Springer.

World Health Organization. (2017). *Communicating risk in public health emergencies.* https://apps.who.int/iris/handle/10665/259807

World Health Organization. (2021). *Framework for strengthening health emergency preparedness in cities and urban settings.* https://www.who.int/publications/i/item/9789240037830

World Health Organization. (2022). *About WHO.* https://www.who.int/about

Figure Credits

Fig. 1: Source: https://www.fema.gov/sites/default/files/documents/fema_ccds-all-sheets.pdf.

Fig. 2: Source: https://www.fema.gov/sites/default/files/2020-04/CPG201Final20180525.pdf.

Fig. 3: Adapted from World Health Organization, Framework for Strengthening Health Emergency Preparedness in Cities and Urban Settings, p. 15. Copyright © 2021 by World Health Organization (WHO).

Fig. 4: Source: https://www.cdc.gov/climateandhealth/effects/default.htm.

Appendix A

Reducing Confusion With Some Critical Terms

The following content provides some basic information and terminology related to public and community health.

Public and Community Health

Public health is the area of health care that focuses on prevention and control of disease and disability, with particular concern for groups (i.e., populations and communities). Healthy behaviors and wellness are important for public health. **Figure A.1** identifies the major core sciences that are associated with public health and used to meet its goals.

Community health focuses on providing comprehensive accessible services to a community to ensure health needs are met and that it considers social determinants of health that affect the community and aims to reduce health disparities while supporting health equity. The latter aim involves an increased emphasis on advocacy and policy development and implementation to ensure a healthy community.

Who Does Public and Community Health Serve?

Within public and community health, various terms are used to identify those who need assistance. Examples of these terms include the following:

- *Individuals* (also *patients*, *clients*, and *consumers*)
- *Families*
- *Aggregates* or *populations*
- *Communities*

The public and community health focus is less on individuals and more on groups (e.g., families; populations, such as persons with heart disease; and communities).

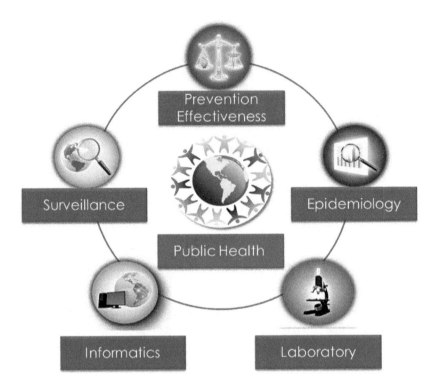

Figure A.1.   Public health core sciences.

Health Care Providers

Health care providers are individuals and organizations providing health services. Examples of individuals are professionals such as physicians, registered nurses, pharmacists, social workers, and others (e.g., nutritionists, government health inspectors [food, business safety], health educators, community planners, epidemiologists, public policymakers, school health staff, community first responders). Health care organizations include acute care hospitals, clinics, community-based service agencies, home health care agencies, centers providing urgent care and emergency services, and pharmacies. In communities, health departments and their associated services, such as clinics and often school health, provide critical services to the community. Within business and industry, occupational health services offer support for employees and health education and prevention and have an impact on the overall health of the community.

Groups and Teams

In this guide, the term *team* is used rather than *group*. Within health care (e.g., acute care, community health, and public health), *team* is more commonly used; staff are members of teams in their workplaces. Students need to become familiar with this term, and to encourage this perspective, the guide refers to student *teams* rather than *groups*.

The Public Health Model

There are three public health core functions:

- **Assessment:** Relates to essential services 1–2
- **Policy development:** Relates to essential services 3–5
- **Assurance:** Relates to essential services 6–10

Nurses who work in public and community health are involved in each of the three core functions and the following 10 public health essential services:

1. Assess and monitor population health status, factors that influence health, and community needs and assets.
2. Investigate, diagnose, and address health problems and hazards affecting the population.
3. Communicate effectively to inform and educate people about health, factors that influence it, and how to improve it.
4. Strengthen, support, and mobilize communities and partnerships to improve health.
5. Create, champion, and implement policies, plans, and laws that impact health.
6. Utilize legal and regulatory actions designed to improve and protect the public's health.
7. Ensure an effective system that enables equitable access to the individual services and care needed to be healthy.
8. Build and support a diverse and skilled public health workforce.
9. Improve and innovate public health functions through ongoing evaluation, research, and continuous quality improvement.
10. Build and maintain a strong organizational infrastructure for public health.

Figure A.2 describes the interrelationship between the core functions and essential services.

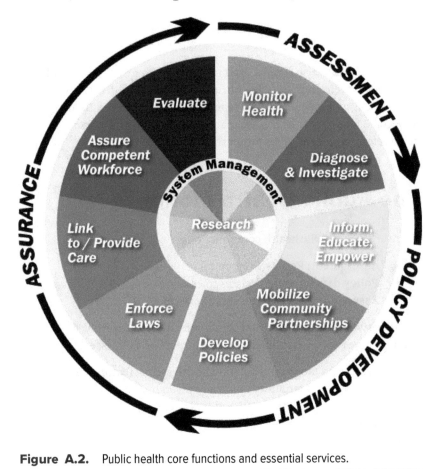

Figure A.2.   Public health core functions and essential services.

Public Health Core Competencies

A collaborative of 24 national organizations concerned with public health education developed the following competencies. These are based on the 10 essential public health services and should be applied to all public health professionals. The goal of this collaboration is to improve public health by ensuring competent staff and effective health care organization performance. Identification of these competencies also recognizes the need for effective coordination and monitoring of outcomes among the key stakeholders in academic institutions, public health practice, and health care communities. Education must include not only preparation education but also ongoing staff education at the work site. The collaboration also notes that there is an ongoing need to develop effective strategies for positive public health outcomes. The following describes the domains—specific activity areas—emphasized in these core competencies (Council on Linkages Between Academia and Public Health Practice, 2021):

Domain 1: Data Analytics and Assessment Skills

Focuses on factors that affect the health of the community, data collection, analysis of data, use of public health informatics applying data and information, assessment of community health status

Domain 2: Policy Development and Program Planning Skills

Development, implementation, and evaluation of policies, programs, and services to improve

Domain 3: Communication Skills

Strategies for internal and external use; responding to information, including misinformation and disinformation; facilitating individual, group, and organization communication

Domain 4: Health Equity Skills

Effective use of principles related to ethics, diversity, equity, inclusion, and justice; self-awareness of biases; working effectively in diverse situations and with diverse people to reduce systematic and structural barriers while advocating for health equity

Domain 5: Community Partnership Skills

Establishing community relationships and working to improve community health and resilience; collaborating and sharing power

Domain 6: Public Health Science Skills

With an understanding of systems, policies, and situations that impact public health, applying the 10 essential public health services, evidence-based practice, and support research to provide more evidence for public health practice

Domain 7: Management and Finance Skills

Effectively applying basic management and finance skills to public health, such as planning, quality, human resources, staff development, finance, policies, integration of diversity, teams and teamwork, collaboration, performance management, using the healthy community model, and application of three public health core functions and 10 essential services

Domain 8: Leadership and Systems-Thinking Skills

Identifies facilitators and barriers related to 10 essential public health services; serves as leader to encourage creativity, innovation, responding to current trends, directing effective change, collaborating with stakeholders in the community, and advocating for public health

Nurses must also follow relevant nursing standards and competencies.

Source: Council on Linkages Between Academia and Public Health Practice. (2021, October). *Core competencies for public health professionals. http://www.phf.org/resourcestools/pages/core_public_health_competencies.aspx*

The nursing profession responded to the development of these public heath core competencies by aligning public health nursing competencies with them. The nursing competencies focus on public health nursing practice, from entry level to senior nursing management positions, and integrate the competencies that were developed for all public health professionals. There are also eight domains in the public health nursing competencies. Given that the focus in this guide is on health equity and disparities, domains that are particularly related to these issues are identified as follows, although many of the other domains are indirectly related to this content (Quad Council Coalition, 2018):

- **Cultural competency skills** focus on understanding and responding to diverse needs, assessing organizational cultural diversity and competence, assessing effects of policies and programs on various populations, and taking action to support a diverse public health workforce (relates to Domain 4).
- **Community dimensions of practice skills** focus on evaluating and developing linkages and relationships within the community, maintaining and advancing partnerships and community involvement, negotiating for the use of community assets, defending public health policies and programs, and evaluating and improving the effectiveness of community engagement (relates to Domain 5).

Source: Quad Council Coalition. (2018). *Community/public health nursing* [C/PHN] *competencies.* *https://www.cphno.org/wp-content/uploads/2020/08/QCC-C-PHN-COMPETENCIES-Approved_2018.05.04_Final-002.pdf*

Public Health Nursing Standards

The American Nurses Association (ANA, 2013) has developed and updated standards for many specialties. *Public Health Nursing: Scope & Standards of Practice* includes standards related to the following: assessment, population diagnosis and priorities, outcomes identification, planning, implementation, coordination of care, health teaching and health promotion, consultation, prescriptive authority, regulatory activities, evaluation, professional performance for public health nursing, ethics, evidence-based practice and research, quality of practice, communication, leadership, collaboration, professional practice evaluation, resource utilization, environmental health, and advocacy. As is true for all ANA standards, and as is mentioned in the guide's content, health equity is an important concern.

Source: American Nurses Association. (2013). *Public health nursing: Scope & standards of practice* (2nd ed.). *https://www.nursingworld.org/nurses-books/public-health-nursing--scope--standards-of-practice-2nd-edition/*

References

American Nurses Association. (2013). *Public health nursing: Scope & standards of practice* (2nd ed.). https://www.nursingworld.org/nurses-books/public-health-nursing--scope--standards-of-practice-2nd-edition/

Council on Linkages Between Academia and Public Health Practice. (2021, October). *Core competencies for public health professionals.* http://www.phf.org/resourcestools/pages/core_public_health_competencies.aspx

Quad Council Coalition. (2018). *Community/public health nursing* [C/PHN] *competencies.* https://www.cphno.org/wp-content/uploads/2020/08/QCC-C-PHN-COMPETENCIES-Approved_2018.05.04_Final-002.pdf

Figure Credits

Fig. A.1: Source: https://www.cdc.gov/training/publichealth101/documents/introduction-to-public-health.pdf.

Fig. A.2: Source: https://www.cdc.gov/publichealthgateway/publichealthservices/originalessentialhealthservices.html.

Appendix B

The National Initiative to Improve the Nation's Health: Healthy People 2030

The U.S. Department of Health and Human Services (HHS), its agencies, and other government departments are responsible for assessing and developing plans and resources to ensure the health of all people who live in the United States by promoting health and preventing disease and illness. The HHS works with health care services at the federal, state, and local levels. As part of this responsibility, Healthy People 2030 is a major federal program that provides a comprehensive plan focused on health promotion and disease prevention and routinely assesses national health status. The initiative is reviewed and updated every 10 years, with five past editions (1979, 1990, 2000, 2010, 2020), and the current edition, which is due to end in 2030. The latest version's vision and major goals focus on the topics of health conditions, health behaviors, populations, settings and systems, and social determinants of health (SDOH).

Health status is determined by measuring birth and death rates, life expectancy, quality of life, morbidity from specific diseases, risk factors, use of ambulatory care and inpatient care, accessibility to health providers and facilities, financing of health care services, health insurance coverage, access to health care, and other factors. Quality is a complex health care issue that affects the health status of individuals and communities. There is not one single factor or behavior that determines outcomes, but rather multiple factors—such as genetics, lifestyle, gender, race/ethnic factors, nutrition, poverty level, education, environment, injury, violence, environment, and unavailability or inaccessibility of quality health services.

Healthy People 2030 Framework

Vision
A society in which all people can achieve their full potential for health and well-being across the life span.

Mission
To promote, strengthen, and evaluate the nation's efforts to improve the health and well-being of all people.

Foundational Principles
Foundational principles explain the thinking that guides decisions about Healthy People 2030:

- Health and well-being of all people and communities are essential to a thriving, equitable society.
- Promoting health and well-being and preventing disease are linked efforts that encompass physical, mental, and social health dimensions.
- Investing to achieve the full potential for health and well-being for all provides valuable benefits to society.
- Achieving health and well-being requires eliminating health disparities, achieving health equity, and attaining health literacy.
- Healthy physical, social, and economic environments strengthen the potential to achieve health and well-being.
- Promoting and achieving the nation's health and well-being is a shared responsibility that is distributed across the national, state, tribal, and community levels, including the public, private, and not-for-profit sectors.
- Working to attain the full potential for health and well-being of the population is a component of decision-making and policy formulation across all sectors.

Overarching Goals

- Attain healthy, thriving lives and well-being, free of preventable disease, disability, injury, and premature death.
- Eliminate health disparities, achieve health equity, and attain health literacy to improve the health and well-being of all.

Office of Disease Prevention and Health Promotion (ODPHP), "Healthy People 2030 Framework," https://health.gov/healthypeople/about/healthy-people-2030-framework, 2021.

- Create social, physical, and economic environments that promote attaining full potential for health and well-being for all.
- Promote healthy development and healthy behaviors and well-being across all life stages.
- Engage leadership, key constituents, and the public across multiple sectors to take action and design policies that improve the health and well-being of all.

Plan of Action

To achieve the health and well-being of all people, relevant stakeholders need to be active partners across the public, private, and nonprofit sectors. Healthy People conducts regular monitoring of the plan's progress. The results are made public on its website.

The Healthy People objectives are developed to meet the overall goals and are based on data and changed as needed during each 10-year cycle. This includes eight broad outcome measures used to assess the program's vision, 355 measurable core public health objectives with 10-year targets and related evidence-based interventions, developmental goals for public health issues with interventions, and research objectives directed at public health issues for which there are no evidence-based interventions.

Healthy People 2030 focuses on individual health and on communities. It describes a healthy community as one that maintains a high quality of life and is productive and safe, provides both treatment and prevention services to all community members, maintains necessary effective infrastructure (e.g., water, energy, roads, transportation, schools, playgrounds, and other services), and maintains a healthy environment (e.g., issues of pollution, such as with air and water). Educational and community-based programs need to focus on preventing disease and injury, promoting and improving health, and enhancing quality of life. This view of a healthy community relates to the SDOH.

To meet Healthy People goals, community programs and services must provide broad access (e.g., in schools, workplaces, health care facilities, and community sites) and offer prevention, monitoring, treatment, and rehabilitation services.

The Healthy People 2030 initiative not only provides a 10-year plan to improve health care in the United States but also monitors and reports on progress by assessing the outcome status of its goals and objectives. Data on current outcomes can be found on the Healthy People website. At the end of the 10-year period, all outcomes are evaluated and summarized. This information is then used to develop the plan for the next 10 years—the goals, objectives, and leading indicators.

Stakeholders

Many organizations, government, and individuals are involved in the development, implementation, and evaluation of the Healthy People initiative. Nurses need to understand the importance of stakeholders so that they can collaborate with relevant stakeholders and advocate for healthy communities. **Figure B.1** describes the Healthy People stakeholders.

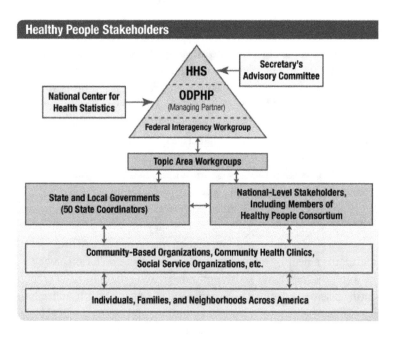

Figure B.1.   Healthy People stakeholders.

Healthy People 2030: Emergency Preparedness

See information about emergency preparedness and updates on this topic at https://health.gov/healthypeople/objectives-and-data/browse-objectives/emergency-preparedness.

Healthy People 2030: Current Information

- Explore the leading health Indicators used by Healthy People to monitor its outcomes.
  Source: https://health.gov/healthypeople/objectives-and-data

- Explore SDOH and relationship to Healthy People.
  Source: https://health.gov/healthypeople/objectives-and-data

- Explore overall health and well-being measures.
  Source: https://health.gov/healthypeople/objectives-and-data

References

U.S. Department of Health and Human Services, Office of Disease Prevention and Health Promotion. (2021a). *Healthy People 2030.* https://health.gov/healthypeople

U.S. Department of Health and Human Services, Office of Disease Prevention and Health Promotion. (2021b). *Tools for action.* https://health.gov/healthypeople/tools-action

Figure Credits

Fig. B.1: Source: https://www.cdc.gov/nchs/about/factsheets/factsheet-hp2030.htm.

Appendix C

Institute of Medicine/National Academy of Medicine Reports

The National Academy of Medicine (NAM) is the former Institute of Medicine (IOM), and since 2015 it has been referred to as NAM. The IOM/NAM has provided significant examination of health care issues and expert advice to health care organizations, individual providers, and health policymakers, both governmental and nongovernmental (NAM, 2021). The IOM/NAM is a nongovernmental, nonprofit organization that was created in 1970. Why is it mentioned in this guide, which deals with equity and disparities? Its reports cover many topics, some of which are relevant to this content. The NAM asks experts to examine an issue, provides staff and funding for the review, and then publishes information from the review and often identifies recommendations (Finkelman, 2017). These recommendations are not laws or regulations, but they often have a major impact on health care decision-making.

The following are brief summaries of early reports that had a significant influence on how the nation's health care delivery system and health policy view quality care as well as more current reports that highlight some areas of interest to this guide's content. Some of the reports are mentioned within the guide's content.

To Err Is Human (**1999**) Due to growing questions about quality care, President William Clinton's Advisory Commission on Consumer Protection and Quality in the Health Care Industry stimulated further examination of quality and asked the IOM to further examine health care, focusing on errors. The report from this request, *To Err Is Human*, stirred a strong reaction by indicating that there were many errors in the U.S. health care system. The results were widely discussed in the media, so consumers became more aware of this problem. In addition, the report emphasized that the health care delivery system put too much emphasis on blame for errors, particularly on individual staff. This led to an active initiative to alter this approach.

Most errors are system errors, not individuals making mistakes. The report focused on acute care.

Crossing the Quality Chasm (2001) A second major report on health care quality followed *To Err Is Human*. It focused on broader issues of quality care and concluded that more information was needed. This report also focused on acute care. Even with President Clinton's commission's review and two extensive reviews and reports on health care quality, there was still concern that we did not know enough and that the problem was extensive. Public and community health also needed to be examined, and later reports included this vital health care area.

Envisioning the National Healthcare Quality Report (2001) The 1999 and 2001 reports mentioned earlier identified the need for systematic monitoring of health care quality to better understand the status of quality care. This monitoring needed to be done routinely and include analysis and recommendations for improvement. *Envisioning the National Healthcare Quality Report* described an initial framework for the new annual monitoring process and report. The Agency for Healthcare Research and Quality, an agency within the HHS, is responsible for this annual report (titled the *National Healthcare Quality and Disparities Report*), which initially focused solely on quality care.

Unequal Treatment: Confronting Racial and Ethnic Disparities in Health Care (2003) This report began to expand the health care perspective by including more about public and community health. As more was learned about quality care, it became clear that there were health disparities due in particular to bias, prejudice, and stereotyping. Just as with the issue of quality care, there was a need to monitor disparities, and this led to the development of a monitoring system and report similar to the *National Healthcare Quality and Disparities Report*, which was later combined with the quality report.

Health Professions Education: A Bridge to Quality (2003) This report moved the quality care discussion to health professions education. With the growing recognition that care needed to improve, which required routine monitoring and improvement, it was determined that a key ingredient to accomplishing this objective was staff—namely whether they were prepared to provide effective and efficient care to diverse populations. This conclusion and the report were critical in that the recommendations included five core competencies that all health care professionals should meet. It is significant that the experts decided to identify competencies that did not focus on one health care profession. These competencies are as follows:

1. Provide patient-centered care (person-centered).
2. Work in interprofessional teams.
3. Employ evidence-based practice.
4. Apply quality improvement.
5. Utilize informatics.

Later, the nursing profession developed core competencies for nursing (Quality and Safety Education for nurses [QSEN]) that related to these core health profession competencies; however, it is important that nursing avoids separating itself from these core competencies. The major difference is that QSEN has six competencies and separates quality from safety, and the IOM/NAM recommendation on core competencies considers safety an integral part of quality (QSEN, 2020).

Health Literacy (**2004**) Aimed at examining diversity and disparities, the report *Health Literacy* recognized that health literacy has a major impact on quality care and the health of individuals and communities.

Health Literacy: A Prescription to End Confusion (**2004**) Communication is critical in health care—both written and oral and with all stakeholders. This includes individuals, families, staff, communities, other professionals, and government, among others. Effective partnerships require effective, ongoing communication. When problems with communication occur, health literacy issues may arise. Understanding is necessary for effective health care decision-making—affecting locations to obtain treatment, treatment providers, types of treatment, the ability to follow treatment, the ability to engage in self-care, questions to ask health care providers, and so on. Yet, millions of Americans cannot understand or act on this information. This report discussed health literacy and methods to improve communication for individuals and populations.

Keeping Patients Safe: Transforming the Work Environment for Nurses (**2004**); **The Future of Nursing: Leading Change, Advancing Health** (**2010**); **The Future of Nursing 2020–2030: Charting a Path to Achieve Health Equity** (**2020**) Some of the IOM/NAM reports have focused on nursing. One of the significant early reports was *Keeping Patients Safe: Transforming the Work Environment for Nurses*, which primarily discussed acute care nursing practice, particularly staff nurses and related workforce issues. In 2010, a landmark report titled *The Future of Nursing: Leading Change, Advancing Health* examined current and future roles of nurses. The third report mentioned is directly related to the content of this guide, *The Future of Nursing 2020–2030: Charting* *a Path to Achieve Health Equity.* These reports are discussed in relevant content in the guide.

The Future of the Public's Health in the 21st Century (2003) and Who Will Keep the Public Healthy? (2003) The initial reports from the IOM focused on acute care, although some of the content could be applied to public and community health. There was slow recognition that separating acute care from public and community health or ignoring the health care delivery system as a whole was not effective. In 2003, this view changed with the publication of two key public and community health reports. *The Future of the Public's Health in the 21st Century* examined the need to apply a population health approach, develop effective public health infrastructure, establish partnerships, ensure accountability, implement evidence-based practice, and utilize clear communication. *Who Will Keep the Public Healthy?* turned the focus to identifying the public health competencies, which are related to informatics, genomics, communication, culture, community-based participatory research, global health, policy and law, and public health ethics. The report provided a guide for public and community health education content, such as for nursing.

Informed Consent and Health Literacy (2015) The *Informed Consent and Health Literacy* report discussed a specific issue related to health literacy, which by 2015 was recognized as a major concern in health care delivery. Participants in research are asked to sign a consent form, and agreeing to do so should be an informed decision. In order to do this, participants must understand the information they are given. Ensuring that participants can agree and understand prior to participating in a research study is a critical part of ethics and participant rights.

Health Literacy: Past, Present, and Future (2015) Given the concern about health literacy, *Health Literacy* examined the problems, origins, and consequences of adult health literacy. Adults who do not have the required level of health literacy may not be able to engage safely in their own health and health care decision-making. The report includes solutions such as the need for organizational changes, including system changes to assist in reducing health literacy.

A Framework for Educating Health Professionals to Address Social Determinants of Health (2016) As more has been learned about the importance of SDOH, there has been growing recognition that health care professionals need to learn about these determinants so that they are more aware of the impact on health and disparities. Professionals will then be better able to intervene and improve the health of individuals, communities, and populations.

Collaboration Between Health Care and Public Health (2016) *Collaboration Between Health Care and Public Health* discussed the need for effective collaboration between acute health care and public health. This partnership needs to include shared goals, community engagement, aligned leadership, sustainability, and data and analysis. There are barriers to this collaboration, including inadequate communication, working with interprofessional teams, understanding diverse cultures, and more, that must be addressed.

Communities in Action: Pathways to Health Equity (2017) *Communities in Action* continues to examine health equity, disparities, and SDOH. It particularly noted that we know individual behavior and health status are important, but there is also a need to view these issues from a community perspective. It is the community that has a strong impact on poverty, unemployment, poor education, inadequate housing, poor public transportation, interpersonal violence, and struggling neighborhoods, all of which influence health. Social policies also make a difference in inequalities and contribute to health inequities. The report examined the causes of and possible solutions to health inequities, emphasizing the importance of communities in promoting health equity.

Perspectives on Health Equity and Social Determinants of Health (2017) *Perspectives on Health Equity and Social Determinants of Health* examined the social factors that influence the nation's health (i.e., SDOH); racism and poverty, which result in inequitable social, environmental, and economic conditions; and health disparities. It included content on policies and strategies used to address these problems, focusing on the need for collective actions.

Community-Based Health Literacy Interventions (2018) *Community-Based Health Literacy Interventions* focused on community interventions to reduce health literacy problems, examining types of community-based literacy interventions, and methods to evaluate their results. It also provided and described examples. Community infrastructure and staff are critical elements to success, as is a commitment to improve community trust.

Immigration as a Social Determinant of Health (2018) The United States has a large immigrant population, which experiences systematic marginalization and discrimination that often results in health disparities. *Immigration as a Social Determinant of Health* examined the relationship between the immigration experience and health outcomes.

Improving Access to and Equity of Care for People With Serious Illness (2019) At the time *Improving access to and Equity of Care for People With Serious Illness* was completed, the CDC estimated that approximately 40 million people in the United States had a serious illness. This type of disease limits daily activities. As health disparities were examined, it was noted that this population also experiences disparities due to race, ethnicity, gender, geography, socioeconomic status, and insurance status. This is found in multiple communities, interfering with health care access and quality. Improvement requires engagement and feedback from individuals (patient and family), health care providers, organizations, and communities.

Integrating Social Care Into the Delivery of Health Care: Moving Upstream to Improve the Nation's Health (2019) With the recognition of the importance of the SDOH in regard to health equity and disparities, the health care delivery system must turn to improvement. The key questions addressed in *Integrating Social Care Into the Delivery of Health Care* were as follows:

- How can services that address social needs be integrated into clinical care?
- What type of infrastructure will be needed to facilitate that integration?

The report concluded that five complementary activities should be used ensure integration of social care into health care: awareness, adjustment, assistance, alignment, and advocacy. The report discussed these activities and stated that they should be used by health care organizations and providers, communities, social services, and governments.

Population Health in Rural America (2020) Rural areas of the United States experience many health problems and difficulties with receiving effective and timely health care. People who live in rural areas are a vulnerable and diverse population. Rural areas also experience serious health care delivery problems, such as a shortage of health care professionals and services.

Population Health in Challenging Times: Insights From Key Domains: Proceedings of a Workshop (2021) *Population Health in Challenging Times* examined population health, which is a complex area of health care. The workshop identified key areas of concern in population health, supporting the recognition that this type of health is a significant issue in the nation's health.

Priorities on the Health Horizon: Informing PCORI's Strategic Plan (2021) This report discussed the need for more evidence to support health care delivery and practice. It particularly focuses on equitable, stakeholder-driven, evidence-guided, patient-centered care. All of this requires effective collaborative relationships between patients, families, clinicians, healthcare administrators, researchers, and policymakers. PCORI is the Patient-Centered Outcomes Research Institute, an independent nonprofit, nongovernmental organization in Washington, DC, that was authorized by Congress in 2010 to address the gap in information needed to make effective health care decisions. (For more information, visit https://www.pcori.org/about/about-pcori.)

Dialogue About the Workforce for Population Health Improvement: Proceedings of a Workshop (2021) A workshop focused on the needs of the population health workforce to improve health produced this report. Some of the discussion topics included peer-to-peer chronic disease management educators, health navigators, community health workers, public and health and health care leaders, developing competencies of the nonmedical and nonpublic health workforce, and application of the health in all policies model.

Exploring the Role of Critical Health Literacy in Addressing the Social Determinants of Health: Proceedings of a Workshop in Brief (2021) Due to the growing concern about the SDOH, a discussion and subsequent report focused on critical health literacy. It particularly addressed the impact of health literacy on SDOH and vulnerable populations. The emphasis was on using literacy strategies to support effective health literacy associated with SDOH.

To Achieve Health Equity, Leverage Nurses and Increase Funding for School and Public Health Nursing (2022) *To Achieve Health Equity, Leverage Nurses and Increase Funding for School and Public Health Nursing* focused on nursing, but rather than discussing acute care, it examined the roles of nursing in public health, driven by the need to improve health equity. Improvements in public health nursing education are needed. The key recommendations are for the next 10 years include these:

- Strengthening nursing education
- Promoting diversity, inclusivity, and equity in nursing education and the workforce

- Investing in school and public health nurses
- Protecting nurses' health and well-being
- Preparing nurses for disaster and public health emergency response
- Increasing the number of PhD-prepared nurses

Reducing Inequalities Between Lesbian, Gay, Bisexual, Transgender, and Queer Adolescents and Cisgender, Heterosexual Adolescents: Proceedings of a Workshop (2022) Lesbian, gay, bisexual, transgender, and queer adolescents and cisgender, heterosexual adolescents are at risk for health and social problems. As a vulnerable population, they require assessment and interventions that address health equity and reduce disparities. This report examined these concerns.

Realizing the Promise of Equity in the Organ Transplantation System (2022) Organ transplantation is a complex health need that is supported by a complex system. A key concern is health equities and disparities for some who need this care. This report discussed the many issues patients and families experience and the system that supports organ transplantation.

Closing Evidence Gaps in Clinical Prevention (2022) This report examined the need for more research to provide evidence supporting effective clinical prevention working in collaboration with the HHS and U.S. Preventive Services Task Force. (For more information, visit https://www.ahrq.gov/cpi/about/otherwebsites/uspstf/index.html.)

Measuring Sex, Gender Identity, and Sexual Orientation (2022) *Measuring Sex, Gender Identity, and Sexual Orientation* explores current information on the topics of sex, gender identity, and sexual orientation. This understanding it is important in appreciating issues related to this population.

Examples of Other Reports

- *School Success: An Opportunity for Population Health* (2019)
- *A Roadmap to Reducing Childhood Poverty* (2019)
- *Virtual Clinical Trials: Challenges and Opportunities* (2019)

NAM publishes many reports annually. Visit the link below to identify current reports.

Access to IOM/NAM Reports

The reports listed and other IOM/NAM resources can be read online or downloaded for free using the guest status. Full or parts of reports can be reviewed. There is no fee to access these reports. This information can be accessed at https://nam.edu/publications/.

References

Finkelman, A. (2017). *Teaching the IOM: Implications of the IOM Reports for Nursing Education* (Vols. 1–2; 4th ed.). American Nurses Association.

QSEN Institute. (2020). *QSEN Institute competencies.* https://qsen.org/competencies/

Index

trauma, 42–44
triage, disaster, 27–28

U

Unequal Treatment: Confronting Racial and Ethnic Disparities in Health Care report, 76–77
United Nations (UN), 17
UN Office for Disaster Reduction (UNDRR), 17
urban areas, and preparedness, 40–41
U.S. Department of Health and Human Services (HHS), 3, 47, 69

V

vulnerable populations, 37–38

W

warning, 24
watch, 24
water crisis, 6
weather-related disasters, 10–11
    and disparities, 5–6
Who Will Keep the Public Healthy? report, 78
World Health Organization (WHO), 16–17, 52

Z

Zika virus, 10

About the Author

Anita Finkelman, MSN, RN is a nurse educator and consultant, currently providing services in the U.S. and Israel, where she has been visiting faculty at Recanati School for Community Health Professions at Ben-Gurion University of the Negev and consulted with several Israeli universities. She served on the nursing faculty at Bouvé College of Health Sciences, School of Nursing, Northeastern University, where she taught undergraduate and graduate online courses and led the nursing school's CCNE accreditation process for undergraduate and graduate programs with full accreditation received. She previously served as an assistant professor of nursing at the University of Oklahoma College of Nursing, where she taught undergraduate and graduate nursing online courses and served as course coordinator for undergraduate nursing research. At the University of Cincinnati, Finkelman was an associate professor of clinical nursing, the director of continuing education, and the director of the undergraduate program (BSN), and taught public/community health, mental health nursing, nursing leadership, health policy, research courses, and clinical practicum. She has worked with several smaller colleges to develop and implement online programs and develop curriculum for pre-licensure nursing students.

Finkelman earned her BSN from Texas Christian University and her master's degree in psychiatric-mental health nursing/clinical nurse specialist from Yale University. She completed post-master's graduate work in healthcare policy and administration at George Washington University and participated as a fellow in the Health Policy Institute at George Mason University. Her nursing experience includes clinical, educational, and administrative positions and considerable experience developing distance education programs and curriculum, as well as a long history of teaching online. Finkelman has extensive management experience serving in various positions in psychiatric-mental health settings (acute care and community), having served as the director of staff education for two acute care hospitals and within clinical nurse specialist positions. As a consultant, she focuses on areas of curriculum and quality improvement, teaching-learning practices, distance education, healthcare administration and policy, nursing education accreditation, and assisting nurses in their publishing endeavors.

She has authored many books, chapters, and journal articles, served on journal editorial boards, and made presentations on nursing education, healthcare administration, health policy, healthcare quality improvement, continuing education, and psychiatric-mental health nursing, both nationally and internationally. She serves as a consultant to publishers in the areas of distance education and product development.

Finkelman's textbooks include *Professional Nursing Concepts* (Jones and Bartlett Learning, 5th ed., 2021); *Quality Improvement: A Guide for Integration in Nursing*, (Jones & Bartlett Learning, 2nd ed., 2020); *Leadership and Management for Nurses: Core Competencies for Quality Care* (Pearson Education, Inc., 4th ed., 2020); and *Case Management for Nurses* (Pearson Education, Inc., 2010). She has also authored chapters in M. Nies and M. McEwen's (Eds.) *Community Health Nursing: Promoting the Health of Aggregates*, Philadelphia, PA: W.B. Saunders Company.

Printed in the USA
CPSIA information can be obtained
at www.ICGtesting.com
LVHW081920050124
768188LV00004B/20